616.994

REGENT COLLEGE

70000038537

WITHDRAWN FROM STOCK

LEARNING RESOURCES CENTRE
REGENT COLLEGE
REGENT ROAD
LEICESTER   LE1 7LW
TELEPHONE: (0116) 255 4629

Return on or before the last date stamped below.

7 DAY
BOOK

KT-514-302

➔ Also available in thefacts series

7 00000 38537

the**facts**

Breast
cancer
SAUNDERS & JASSAL

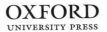

OXFORD
UNIVERSITY PRESS

OXFORD
UNIVERSITY PRESS

Great Clarendon Street, Oxford OX2 6DP

Oxford University Press is a department of the University of Oxford.
It furthers the University's objective of excellence in research, scholarship,
and education by publishing worldwide in

Oxford New York

Auckland Cape Town Dar es Salaam Hong Kong Karachi
Kuala Lumpur Madrid Melbourne Mexico City Nairobi
New Delhi Shanghai Taipei Toronto

With offices in

Argentina Austria Brazil Chile Czech Republic France Greece
Guatemala Hungary Italy Japan Poland Portugal Singapore
South Korea Switzerland Thailand Turkey Ukraine Vietnam

Oxford is a registered trade mark of Oxford University Press
in the UK and in certain other countries

Published in the United States
by Oxford University Press Inc., New York

© Oxford University Press 2009

The moral rights of the authors have been asserted
Database right Oxford University Press (maker)

First edition published 2009

All rights reserved. No part of this publication may be reproduced,
stored in a retrieval system, or transmitted, in any form or by any means,
without the prior permission in writing of Oxford University Press,
or as expressly permitted by law, or under terms agreed with the appropriate
reprographics rights organization. Enquiries concerning reproduction
outside the scope of the above should be sent to the Rights Department,
Oxford University Press, at the address above

You must not circulate this book in any other binding or cover
and you must impose this same condition on any acquirer

British Library Cataloguing in Publication Data

Data available

Typeset in Plantin
by Cepha Imaging Pvt. Ltd., Bangalore, India
Printed in Great Britain on acid-free paper by Ashford Colour Press Ltd, Gosport, Hampshire

ISBN 9780199558698

10 9 8 7 6 5 4 3 2 1

Whilst every effort has been made to ensure that the contents of this book are as complete, accurate
and up-to-date as possible at the date of writing, Oxford University Press is not able to give any
guarantee or assurance that such is the case. Readers are urged to take appropriately qualified
medical advice in all cases. The information in this book is intended to be useful to the general
reader, but should not be used as a means of self-diagnosis or for the prescription of medication.

Contents

Abbreviations

ADH	atypical ductal hyperplasia
ALH	atypical lobular hyperplasia
BSE	breast self-examination
CT	computed tomography
DCIS	ductal carcinoma *in situ*
DVT	deep venous thrombosis
ER	oestrogen receptors
FNA	fine needle aspiration
GnRH	gonadotrophin-releasing hormone analogues
Her2	human epidermal growth factor receptor
HRT	hormone replacement therapy
IVF	*in vitro* fertilization
LCIS	lobular carcinoma *in situ*
LH	luteinizing hormone
LVI	lympho-vascular invasion
MRI	magnetic resonance imaging
NSAIDs	non-steroidal anti-inflammatory drugs
PgR	progesterone receptors
SNB	sentinel lymph node biopsy
TRAM	trans-rectus abdominis muscle
VEGF	vascular endothelial growth factor

1

Breasts and breast cancer

➡ Key Points

- Most women will experience symptoms in their breasts at some time in their life, and the vast majority will be due to a benign cause.
- Women should always consult their doctor if a symptom persists and is of concern.
- Cancer occurs when cells grow abnormally and invade parts of the body.
- Breast cancer affects around 1 in 8 women in developed countries.
- Breast cancer can occur in men, however this is very rare.

Breast cancer is one of the most common cancers affecting women in the Western world and is continuing to increase in frequency. Whilst it is predominantly a disease of older women, it can and does occur in women under 30 years of age. Most people will know of someone who has faced breast cancer. This, along with the emphasis in the media, places breast cancer in the minds of all of us and it may be a source of fear for many women—not just those who actually develop the disease.

A greater focus on this health issue in both the scientific world as well as the general public has facilitated great advances in the detection and treatment of breast cancer. Breast screen programmes, dedicated breast clinics, modern treatments and vigorous ongoing research are all playing their part in improving the chances of successful treatment and, in some cases, avoiding breast cancer in the first place. However, with this focus has also come a tendency towards misinformation, with many people having an incomplete understanding of the issues surrounding breast cancer.

This book aims to provide a balanced guide to breast cancer for all women, as well as their partners, sons, fathers, brothers and whoever else has an interest in learning more about this complex problem.

Whilst breast cancer is a serious and potentially life-threatening condition, most breast symptoms do not mean cancer, and when a diagnosis of cancer is made, the treatments and outcomes are frequently not as severe as imagined. There is a trend away from removal of the breast (mastectomy). Newer, more effective treatments are continually being developed and these modern treatments offer women, particularly with early breast cancers, a real chance of cure.

Breast disease

Whilst breast cancer is common, most breast symptoms will not culminate in a diagnosis of cancer. However, early detection of breast cancer is paramount to offering the very best chance of cure and as such, it is important for women to seek medical attention should they develop any breast complaint. It is sad to think that some women who delay seeing a doctor for fear of what might be revealed are actually compromising their chances of getting the best treatment.

> Most breast symptoms are not due to cancer but it is important to report any persisting change to a doctor.

Breast symptoms may include a lump, breast pain (mastalgia) and skin or nipple changes such as infection, ulceration or discharge. Evaluation of most of these complaints will lead to diagnosis of a benign problem, often without the need for any surgery. Occasionally, surgery will be required when a diagnosis has not been otherwise possible. This will usually consist of removing a small piece of breast tissue (a biopsy) under general anaesthetic to get a clearer idea of what is going on. For most benign conditions, medical follow up will not be necessary. With other benign conditions, there may be an increased risk of cancer in the future and as such the doctor may recommend some form of monitoring such as an annual mammogram.

When a diagnosis of cancer is made, the doctor will go through the diagnosis carefully and may involve other doctors such as a surgeon. As mentioned above, surgery does not necessarily mean mastectomy. In any case, modern techniques place a strong emphasis on achieving good cosmetic outcomes whilst not compromising the cancer treatment. The surgeon will discuss all of the options and the pros and cons of each. When surgery is appropriate, women will have a clear idea of what is to happen prior to being anaesthetized (see Chapter 8).

The breast—some basic facts
Function

The primary purpose of the breast is to produce milk for a newborn baby. This is done using a series of milk glands, which drain via an interconnected duct structure up to the nipple. These milk glands are usually lying dormant within the breast fat but become modified for use. At this time, the breast is fuller and firmer as the milk glands become more prominent relative to the surrounding fat.

Most women will also notice changes in their breasts related to their monthly cycle. All of these changes are, in the main, controlled by hormones such as oestrogen, progesterone, and prolactin. The naturally changing breast can make monitoring and detection of disease more difficult—another reason why careful medical assessment should be sought for any concerns.

Breasts also play an important role in a woman's self image. They are a powerful symbol of femininity, motherhood and in many cultures, sexuality. It is critical to consider these issues in any discussion about treatment for breast disease.

Men have a basic form of breast—identical to the female breast prior to its development in puberty when it becomes primed for pregnancy and breast-feeding. Whilst male breasts can develop cancers and other conditions, these are rare occurrences, particularly when compared with the frequency of breast disease in women.

Anatomy

The breast is predominantly fatty tissue. As mentioned, milk glands and ducts lie within this tissue. The breast is enclosed within a thin fibrous envelope, which separates it from the skin above and the muscle underneath.

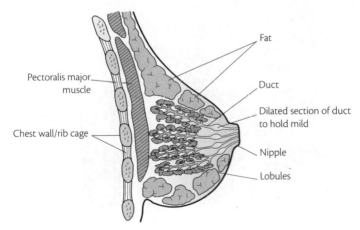

Fat

Pectoralis major muscle

Duct

Dilated section of duct to hold mild

Chest wall/rib cage

Nipple

Lobules

Figure 1.1 The structure of the breast.

Fibrous bands or ligaments run through the breast, maintaining the shape of the fibrous envelope. It is these ligaments which stretch under the influence of gravity as a woman ages, leading to a natural 'sag'. Breasts also tend to 'thin out' over the years as the milk-producing glands become less prominent and are replaced with fat. This can make detection of disease easier as abnormalities are easier to feel as well as see on a mammogram.

The breast sits on the chest lying over ribs and muscles. Immediately under the breast is the pectoralis major muscle and beneath that, the pectoralis minor muscle. Traditionally these muscles were removed in breast cancer surgery, however this is almost never done these days.

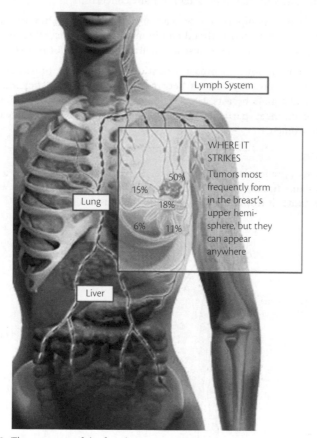

Figure 1.2 The anatomy of the female upper torso.

Blood is supplied from both the armpit region (the axillary artery and vein) as well as from blood vessels within the rib cage (the internal mammary artery and vein). When present, breast cancer cells can spread via these blood vessels to other sites within the body such as the lungs, liver and bones where new tumours can grow—these are metastases.

Another important consideration in breast anatomy is the lymphatic system. This is a network of vessels and glands throughout the body, which instead of carrying blood—like arteries and veins—carry lymph. Lymph is fluid left behind in the body's tissues by blood vessels. Its purpose is to bathe the cells and facilitate transfer of nutrients and waste back and forth. It is collected by lymphatic vessels, which filter through a series of stations—lymph glands/ nodes—on their way to delivering the fluid back into the blood system. Lymph nodes are typically kidney bean-shaped structures, less than 1cm in size. They purify lymph of bacteria and other harmful substances, including cancer cells, before the lymph drains back into the blood system. Lymph nodes may swell in size when there is work to do, such as dealing with a nearby infection. Many people would have experienced this with, for example, neck gland swelling with a sore throat.

As with blood vessels, lymphatics can facilitate cancer spread. Cancer cells break off the original tumour and may be picked up by lymphatics, thus travelling to nearby lymph nodes and sometimes beyond to more distant lymph nodes. The nodes may increase in size as they fight and/or become occupied by these invading cells as new colonies of cancer cells grow. Thus, it is important to have an understanding of where the breast's lymphatics travel so as to be able to assess the relevant lymph nodes for cancer.

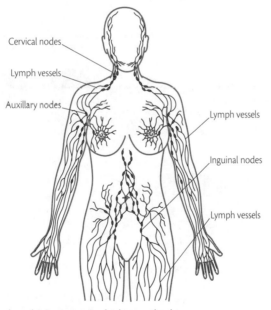

Figure 1.3 The lymphatic system in the human body.

The breast's lymphatic vessels typically drain from the nipple outwards through the breast to lymph nodes in the armpit (the axilla; thus they are called axillary nodes) on that side. From there, lymph will pass to the nodes above the collarbone (supraclavicular nodes) and on into the neck and chest. Sometimes, the lymphatics may travel instead from the breast to nodes behind the breastbone—the internal mammary nodes. Many breast cancer operations will target the axillary nodes as well as the breast in an attempt to more fully remove the cancer. This will be discussed further in Chapter 8.

So what is cancer?

Cancer is a term which covers an incredibly diverse range of conditions which can potentially affect any part of the human body. The characteristic feature shared by all cancers is that the usual balance between cell multiplication and cell death is lost. Whilst cells all over our bodies are damaged regularly, our immune system will usually either repair or destroy them. If for some reason a cell becomes resistant to these control mechanisms, it may start multiplying out of control—a tumour is born. It is not likely to be one error within the body which leads to a tumour but more commonly a series of failures which leads to the problem.

> The characteristic feature of cancer is that the usual balance between cell multiplication and cell death is lost.

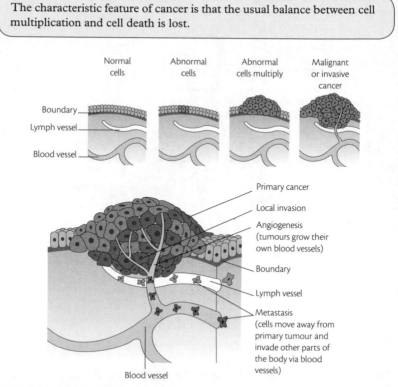

Figure 1.4 What is cancer?

Tumours, or neoplasms, as they are sometimes called, can be benign or malignant. Benign tumours are those which, whilst growing in an uncontrolled fashion, are unable to spread beyond the confines in which they have arisen. As such, they rarely cause life-threatening problems, unless via their growth they press on an important neighbouring structure. Benign brain tumours can cause problems this way; however, within the breast, benign tumours are not dangerous. Malignant tumours, by contrast, are those which have the ability to spread beyond their immediate anatomical boundaries. They do this by invading into neighbouring structures and also into lymphatic and blood vessels from where they can spread to distant spots as discussed above. It is the invasive component of malignant tumours which gives them the ability to become life-threatening as they spread through the body. The term invasive cancer is another way of describing a malignant tumour.

Survival statistics

♦ Up to 1 in 8 women in developed counties will be diagnosed with breast cancer, most commonly in the over-50 age group.

♦ Modern detection and treatment of breast cancer offers a much greater chance of successful treatment than ever before—over 80% of patients survive long term.

♦ Recent data show that about 86% of women aged over 45 years at diagnosis will be alive after 5 years.

♦ For women diagnosed when they are younger than 45 years survival is lower—an estimated 81% will be alive after 5 years.

Medical jargon

A common source of confusion between doctors and their patients has always been the use of medical terms. Whilst they are part of everyday language for medical professionals, for most non-medical people these terms do little to contribute to the understanding of a difficult topic at what may be a very stressful time. In this book, we have attempted to keep things as simple as possible so as to reach out to a broad cross-section of people from everyday women, to those affected by breast cancer, to concerned relatives and also to health care professionals. Where relevant we have explained the meanings of common terms used and have also included a glossary at the book's conclusion to further reinforce some common meanings.

2

Who is at risk?

> ## ⮕ Key Points
>
> Factors which lead to an increased risk of breast cancer in women:
> - Multiple close family members with breast and/or ovarian cancer aged younger than 50 years at diagnosis
> - A previous benign breast biopsy showing atypia
> - Use of hormone replacement therapy (HRT)
> - Excessive alcohol consumption
> - Being overweight or obese, especially after menopause
> - Some ethnic groups such as Ashkenazi Jewish women

We know that up to 1 in 8 women in 'Western' countries will develop breast cancer over their lifetime, but is there any way we can identify who will be that one, or who will be the 7 out of 8 women who will never get a cancer? Moreover, can we tell *when* a woman is likely to get breast cancer? Finally, is there anything a woman can do to lessen her chances of getting the disease?

Cancer is a kind of degenerative disease—it comes about when the checks and balances which normally make cells grow and die in an orderly fashion get disrupted and our body's immune system can no longer repair or destroy abnormal cells. In fact, our body's cells are constantly being exposed to potentially harmful outside influences such as radiation (which includes sunlight) and toxins in food, which damage cells and potentially lead to cancerous changes. Usually these are repaired by sophisticated cell mechanisms, but as we age we are less able to repair the damage caused by these toxins and so cancer and other illnesses become more common.

> **So the major cause of breast cancer is getting older – and breast cancer is more common as women get older.**

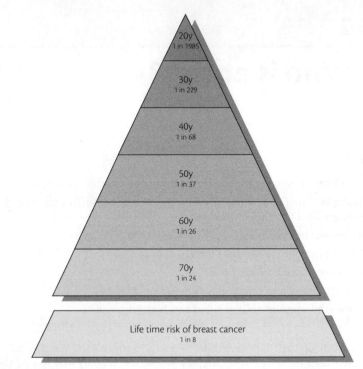

20y
1 in 1985

30y
1 in 229

40y
1 in 68

50y
1 in 37

60y
1 in 26

70y
1 in 24

Life time risk of breast cancer
1 in 8

Figure 2.1 The probability of a woman developing breast cancer within the next 10 years.

Family history

Having a member of the family with a history of breast cancer is very common—some women will have one or two female relatives (such as cousins or aunts) who have had breast cancer. This may put a woman at a slightly higher risk, and these women may be recommended to have annual mammograms.

About 1% of the population however have the odds stacked much higher against them—these are people who come from families where there is a defect in one of a number of genes which make it much more likely a person from these families will develop breast (and/or ovarian) cancer. The commonest of these are known as the *BRCA1* and *BRCA 2* genes. Typically these families will have four or five female members (and occasionally male) who have developed breast or ovarian cancer, and usually at a young age, often under 40 years. The link with ovarian cancer is important—in some families the women have developed ovarian rather than breast cancer. This is also important because ovarian cancer is often a much more deadly disease which may not manifest itself until it is quite advanced, so women from these families need to be aware of how they can decrease their risk of developing this. Figure 2.2 illustrates one such family.

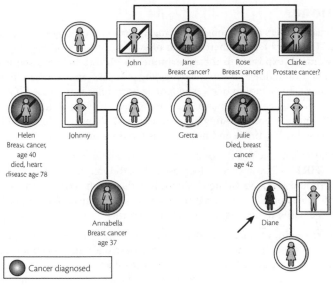

John
Jane
Breast cancer?
Rose
Breast cancer?
Clarke
Prostate cancer?

Helen
Breast cancer,
age 40
died, heart
disease age 78
Johnny
Gretta
Julie
Died, breast
cancer
age 42

Annabella
Breast cancer
age 37
Diane

Cancer diagnosed

Figure 2.2 A family history of breast cancer.

Over the last decade doctors and family members have started to recognize the patterns in these families and members can be referred to specialist doctors in family cancer or genetic clinics. Some families can be offered blood tests which may pick up these gene mutations, so individuals in the family can be tested to see if they carry them—if they do they are much more likely to develop cancer and can look at strategies to minimize or prevent this (see below) and if they do not they can be reassured they are not at increased risk. However, testing will not detect all defective genes and not all families can be tested. It is estimated that around 5% of women who get breast cancer will have one of these genes— particularly if they are less than 40 years old at diagnosis.

Some ethnic groups have a much higher rate of these gene faults, for example people of Ashkenazi Jewish descent.

It is important that a woman brings any concerns about family history to the attention of a doctor.

Benign breast disease

Another factor which may make a woman at a higher risk of breast cancer is having a kind of benign breast disease called atypical ductal (or lobular) hyperplasia—this is diagnosed at biopsy (*not* on a mammogram), and these women should probably have an annual mammogram. Conditions such as simple cysts and fibroadenomas do not put a woman at higher risk of breast cancer, nor are they likely to develop into breast cancers.

Hormones

Many breast cancers are responsive to female hormones oestrogen and progesterone (see Chapter 11), and there is a lot of evidence from studying populations that a woman's exposure to these hormones, both due to those she makes in her own body and due to hormone drugs she may take, may increase the risk of breast cancer. Exposure to one's own female hormones is increased if a woman starts her periods early and has a late menopause. Having children later in life (over 30) and not breastfeeding also increase risk. However, for an individual this increased risk is tiny—and not very easy to do much about!

Taking hormones such as the oral contraceptive pill and hormone replacement therapy (HRT) will also slightly increase risk, although the Pill has such a small effect it should not stop women using this if they wish. HRT used for a short (under 5 years) period to combat menopause symptoms is fairly safe, but any woman is advised to discuss this with her doctor.

Being overweight, at least after the menopause, also increases risk and this is probably because these women make more oestrogen in their body fat once their ovaries shut down. There has been controversy over whether termination of pregnancy increases a woman's risk of breast cancer but there is no evidence whatsoever to suggest this is so.

Alcohol and diet

Excess alcohol (defined as more than two glasses of wine a day or the equivalent) may somewhat increase breast cancer risk. Although much has been written about diet over the years, overall no studies have shown that a particular diet increases or decreases risk. It was once thought that a high intake of soy products may be protective against breast cancer, but there is not much evidence to support this.

Exercise

Regular exercise can reduce the risk of developing breast cancer: it is recommended that people have at least 30 minutes a day of some kind of exercise that makes them a bit breathless. After breast cancer exercise also increases the chance of disease not coming back. It is not understood exactly how this works, but it is probably due to a combination of hormonal influences of exercise and weight control, and its positive influence on the immune system.

Geography

Women from some parts of the world rarely get breast cancer—it seems to be a disease of developed countries such as Western Europe, North America and Australia, although it is rapidly increasing where wealth is increasing, for example in India and Eastern Europe. This is probably because a whole mixture of the risk factors above are coming into play: women are living long enough to get the disease, are starting their periods earlier, having fewer children, taking hormones and getting fatter!

It is interesting to look at the risk of breast cancer in women who are born and brought up in, for example, Japan (very low risk) compared to their descendents who emigrate to the West and *their* descendents who are born and brought up in the West: slowly their risk increases till it becomes Western.

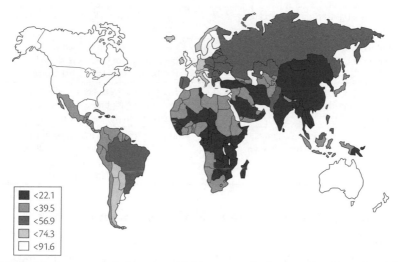

■	<22.1
■	<39.5
■	<56.9
■	<74.3
□	<91.6

Figure 2.3 Breast cancer incidence worldwide: age-standardized rates (world population). Adapted from Ferlay J, Bray F, Pisani P, Parkin DM (2001) *GLOBOCAN 2000: Cancer Incidence, Mortality and Prevalence Worldwide.* IARC Cancer Base No. 5. [1.0] Lyon, France: IARC 2001.

Figure 2.3 illustrates the geographical areas of the world with the highest number of newly diagnosed cases of breast cancer (shown in white) and the geographical areas with the lowest number of newly diagnosed cases (shown in dark gray).

Other risk factors

A few other rare factors significantly increase a woman's chance of getting breast cancer. Previous radiotherapy, especially for Hodgkin's lymphoma, greatly increases the risk. Excessive exposure to radiation, for example a lot of computed tomography (CT) scans as a child, may also increase risk a little.

Are some occupations associated with increased risk? We do not know for sure although there is some suggestion that shift work may slightly increase risk due possibly to it causing hormonal imbalance. Research is currently looking at whether exposure to pesticides at work may also put women at risk.

Table 2.1 Myths about breast cancer risk

Myth	Verdict
Breast cancer can be caused by an injury to the breast—a fall or a knock.	Injury does NOT cause cancer but may draw the woman's attention to a lump.
Deodorants and anti-perspirants contain toxins which increase breast cancer risk.	There is NO evidence that deodorants cause breast cancer.
Wearing a tight-fitting bra will cause breast cancer.	Tight-fitting bras DO NOT cause breast cancer.
Women with larger breasts have a higher risk of developing cancer.	Risk will increase in women who are overweight but breast size alone has not been shown to be a risk factor.
Mammograms can cause breast cancer by 'squeezing' the breast or radiation exposure.	Mammography is safe and effective in screening for breast cancer. See Chapter 4 for further information.
Women with silicone breast implants are not able to have a mammogram.	Implants can make mammography slightly more difficult but it is still both possible and a very effective way of screening for breast cancer.

What can decrease the risk of developing breast cancer?

In general we know that a healthy balanced diet, moderating alcohol intake, maintaining weight at a recommended level and regular exercise of around 30 minutes a day, will decrease the chances of developing both breast cancer and many other diseases. Minimizing HRT use to as short a time as is warranted (suggested as less than 5 years use), and only for the time a woman is getting menopause symptoms such as hot flushes, will also minimize risk.

Having regular screening mammograms will not decrease a woman's chance of developing breast cancer but will increase the likelihood it will be discovered at a very early stage, thus improving the chance of cure and giving her more options for treatment such as lumpectomy rather than mastectomy. Mammography in higher risk women may be recommended to be performed at more frequent intervals—usually every year. For very high risk women it has been shown that magnetic resonance imaging (MRI) of the breast may be the most accurate way to pick up cancers at an early stage. However, this is not widely available (and indeed needs to be done as part of an integrated surveillance programme that includes specialist assessment and mammography). For young women under 50 it may be useful to add an annual breast ultrasound to a screening mammogram.

For women at moderate to high increased risk, there are a number of studies going on around the world to determine if using a drug such as Tamoxifen or Anastrazole can decrease risk—at present these are only routinely available to prevent cancer in a few countries (including the United States) but women can find out about the studies from the websites listed at the end of the book.

For women who fall into a very high risk category, mainly due to a very strong family history or those who have a proven gene mutation, the only established option to decrease breast cancer risk is to consider surgery. Surgery to remove the ovaries (oophorectomy) in pre-menopausal women will decrease breast cancer risk by around 50%—probably by decreasing female hormone exposure. Obviously this has the downside of leading to loss of fertility and menopause. Surgery to remove the breasts (a bilateral prophylactic mastectomy) will decrease a woman's chance of developing breast cancer to virtually zero, but is obviously a difficult and individual decision. If a woman does decide on this option, breast reconstruction can be carried out and this is discussed in detail in Chapter 8.

Table 2.2 Strategies to decrease the risk of developing breast cancer for women who are at an average or high risk

Average risk	High risk
Balanced diet and moderate alcohol	As for average risk women plus consider:
Healthy weight and exercise	◆ Trialling prevention medications
Minimize HRT use	◆ Prophylactic surgery
Regular screening mammograms	◆ Regular high-risk screening with a physical exam, mammograms and MRI

How to assess personal risk

A number of groups around the world have developed computer programmes to help determine an individual's risk of breast cancer. Most of these take into account family history, ethnic origins, plus or minus a past history of breast disease and 'hormonal' risk factors such as age at childbirth. There are websites which can help determine personal risk.

Risk also changes with age. As a woman gets older *without* having developed cancer she is less likely to develop it over the rest of her lifetime.

These risks are based on data drawn from large populations and none can be entirely predictive for an individual—even women who have a gene which predisposes to the disease will not necessarily develop breast cancer. In fact only 50–80% of women with a *BRCA1* or *BRCA2* gene will, and we do not yet know why this is—perhaps it is an interaction of exposure to some toxin in the environment plus the gene fault, or perhaps it is due to a combination of gene changes.

> **Question to ask your doctor: How can I get a gene test?**
>
> *You need to be referred to a genetic or family cancer clinic to have your risk assessed and to discuss all the options.*

This difficulty in assessing an individual's risk means it is best that a woman discusses this with an expert—preferably in a genetic or family cancer clinic. In addition the doctors and counsellors in such a clinic can go over many other issues ranging from confirming family histories to how a gene test is done, what the implications of the results are and how this may impact both physically, emotionally and even financially on a woman and her family.

📄 Case study

Emily is a 43 year old woman who goes to her General Practitioner to discuss her concerns regarding breast cancer. She has never had any breast problems but her sister was diagnosed with breast cancer 2 months previously at the age of 45 and her aunt on her mother's side died following breast cancer some years before when in her 60s. Emily has never had any previous mammograms. Her GP cannot find anything on checking her breasts, and notes she is still getting regular periods having had her second baby 3 years prior – she had her first baby at age 37.

She goes on to have a screening mammogram which is normal but is keen to be assessed by a specialist so is sent to the local family cancer clinic.

The doctor at this clinic takes a detailed family history – Emily is one of 2 sisters, and her mother was one of only 2 sisters. Her maternal grandmother died of what Emily believed was an obstructed bowel in her early 60s (some 20 years ago). The specialist is able to obtain the medical records of Emily's grandmother. These confirm she in fact had ovarian cancer which caused her bowel obstruction and death. Emily meanwhile has discovered that her grandmother had 3 sisters, 2 of whom may have had breast cancer.

This means Emily is potentially at high risk of breast cancer - there may be a gene defect in the family which she may have inherited. Her sister consents to undergo testing for this and is found indeed to carry a *BRCA 1* mutation – her sister then goes on to have both breast and ovaries removed. Emily is tested for the mutation and is found to NOT carry it, so is reassured she can just have routine breast screening.

3

What to look for?

➜ Key Points

◆ Being 'Breast Aware' can be an important part of detecting cancer early.

◆ Medical advice should be sought when breast changes are detected. These include:

Breast lump, thickening or hardening

Dimpling, tethering or flaking of the skin

Nipple change, including retraction, inversion or discharge

Breast pain or soreness

Any change in appearance of the breasts.

◆ Medical assessment will reveal most women's concerns to be of a normal or benign nature.

◆ If you detect a change, seek prompt medical advice but do not panic.

It's a common catch-cry: 'Be Breast Aware'… 'Practice Breast Self-Examination' (BSE). In reality though, many, if not most women, do not regularly examine their breasts. The prevailing notion is that it's too hard to pick up any serious changes when the breasts are lumpy anyway and are constantly changing in relation to the woman's cycle. It is true that breasts are always changing under the influence of menstrual hormones. In addition, some breasts are just lumpier than others. Neither of these issues equates with breast disease nor any increased risk of breast cancer, but they do make breast self-examination more challenging.

Breast awareness

What is breast awareness? It means being comfortable with one's own breasts; their typical appearance, how they feel, and the ways in which they change over the course of a menstrual cycle and as we age. It's when a woman is used to what her breasts are doing in a normal fashion that the abnormal starts to stand out. For women with difficult breasts to monitor—those which are generally 'lumpy' or 'constantly changing'—personal breast awareness, ironically, becomes even more crucial. Who better to pick up subtle changes in such breasts: their owner, or a doctor who might be examining them for the very first time?

Clearly, breast awareness is not a stand-alone tool in the fight against breast cancer. However, along with appropriate medical surveillance, it gives a woman her best chance of detecting a cancer early and in turn, achieving curative treatment.

Breast self-examination

The majority of breast cancers are still detected by a woman herself. This is despite advances in breast screening, increased doctor awareness and all of the sophisticated tests we have at our disposal. However, it has now clearly been shown that ritual monthly self-examination for the majority of women does not lead to increased detection of cancerous breast lumps but *does* lead to excess concerns and investigations of what turn out ultimately (often after surgical biopsy) to be benign changes.

Question to ask our doctor: What is the best way to be breast aware?

Women should be aware of how their normal breasts look and feel. On occasion women should examine themselves as explained in the picture below. However, women should be careful not to become unduly worried about their breasts.

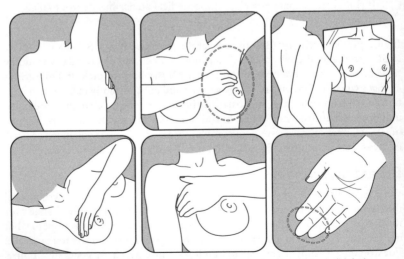

Figure 3.1 A step-by-step illustration of breast self-examination: (a) look; (b) feel.

There are two parts to breast self-examination:

1. *LOOK.* Use a mirror to check the breasts for any changes. In particular, look for changes on the skin: colour, pulling or dents, dimpling, a lump may even be visible bulging through the skin. In addition, look for nipple changes such as retraction or inversion, dryness or even mild ulceration. The inspection should be done in various positions such as leaning forward, hands pushing in on the hips and arms in the air. The idea of changing positions is to increase the chance of seeing something unusual. Compare the breasts. They should look fairly similar.

2. *FEEL.* The shower is a good place to run the hand over each breast. Water and soap make this easier and may enhance detection of lumps. Feel with the flat of the palm and fingers the breast for areas that differ to the rest—it may be a lump, an area of thickening, a band of hard tissue, a tender area. Remember to feel all parts of the breast including under the nipple and up into the armpit. Again, compare the breasts. They should feel fairly similar.

> **Women can start being breast aware and practising breast examination from their 20s or 30s onwards.**

It has been argued that through breast self-examination, some women may develop a false sense of reassurance and avoid medical assessment. Clearly, self-examination is not a substitute for a medical check-up or special tests which doctors may recommend to certain groups. Similarly, breast self-examination can be of little benefit if a woman is not prepared to act on her findings or concerns. Unfortunately, some women will delay seeking medical advice upon detection of an abnormality. This may be for one of many reasons including fear of a cancer diagnosis, denial of the problem or some cultural sensitivity. It is not uncommon to see a woman for the first time in a breast clinic with an already advanced cancer, which may have been obvious to her for some time.

Finally, breast self-examination should not be a trigger for undue anxiety. It is simply a basic way of assessing the breasts that any woman can do. Finding something 'abnormal' does not equate with cancer. Indeed, most breast concerns which women seek medical advice for will turn out to be either part of the 'normal' breast or a benign (non-cancerous) problem.

When is breast self-examination not enough?

Whilst being breast aware is an excellent starting point for all women, in some groups for whom breast cancer risk is higher a programme of regular medical assessment, which may include mammogram, ultrasound or MRI (magnetic resonance imaging), will also be used. This has already been discussed in Chapter 2. The most obvious risk factor for breast cancer, which affects all women, is increasing age. As such, as women get older, it becomes more likely that their doctor will recommend a regular medical check-up as well as some form of radiological imaging—most commonly a mammogram. Many countries now have government-sponsored mammogram screening programmes for women of certain age groups and we will discuss this further in the next chapter.

📄 Case study

Emma is only 26 years old and had never really thought about examining her breasts. However one day she was reading a magazine – in fact the 'Pink' edition of a popular Women's monthly magazine published for Breast Cancer Awareness month.

This explained how to examine breasts and what to look for. After her next period she tried the breast self examination and immediately felt a lump in the upper outer area of her left breast. This was a smooth lump about the size of a small grape which moved about under her fingers. She felt it again over the next few weeks – it did not seem to change with her menstrual cycle and did not go away.

So the next month Emma went to her GP and reported the lump. Her GP thought it felt benign, but still ordered some tests – an ultrasound and a needle biopsy. These confirmed it was a completely benign lump (a *fibroadenoma*) and her GP reassured her that as long as it was so small it would do no harm and she did not need any treatment.

Emma continued to examine herself occasionally and was happy to find no other changes – and the lump she knew was benign never changed.

4

Screening for breast cancer in the population

> ## ➔ Key Points
>
> ◆ Mammograms are an effective way to detect early breast cancer—they are very safe, are well tolerated, are cheap to perform and will detect up to 85% of breast cancers.
>
> ◆ The chance of a mammogram causing cancer is less than 1 in a million.
>
> ◆ Depending on your age, mammograms should be repeated every one to three years.
>
> ◆ Mammographic screening programmes are targeted at women aged 50–69 years but may have some benefit for women aged 40–49 years and above 70 years.

Treatment for breast cancer is ever-improving. Detection of the cancer early in its course, however, remains central to ensuring the highest chance of a cure. It is clear that breast self-examination alone is not enough to achieve this. With the use of additional medical testing, our ability to detect cancers earlier is much enhanced. Research tells us that mammogram screening programmes—directed at specific age groups of women within the population where the risk of cancer is highest—are a highly effective way of bringing about early detection of breast cancer. Most importantly, this translates into better long-term survival rates after treatment.

Mammography

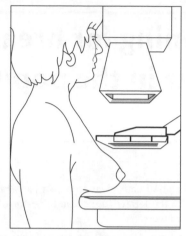

Figure 4.1 An illustration of a mammogram.

This is another way of describing a breast X-ray. The breast is compressed between metallic plates between which the X-ray beams travel. Two or three different angles may be taken and in some situations, focused views on particular areas of concern may be requested. The X-ray pictures can be developed almost instantly, although reading them can take a little more time and is best done by two radiologists trained in breast imaging.

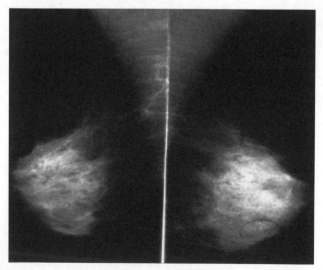

Figure 4.2 Mammogram X-ray images.

Benign lumps are typically rounded and smooth edged. Cancers, by contrast, may be denser in the middle with an irregular edge. The surrounding breast tissue may be distorted by the cancerous invasion. Sometimes, cancerous change may be associated with clusters of calcium flecks which show up on a mammogram as bright white dots. These have a different appearance to the calcium spots of benign change and constitute a powerful way by which early cancerous change can be detected via mammogram.

Mammogram screening

Mammogram screening refers to the process of selecting a certain group of women who are considered to be at risk of breast cancer and performing regular mammograms on all of them, irrespective of whether they have any breast concerns or not. The benefit of this in detecting early breast cancers is most strongly seen in women over 50. There is also some evidence that screening from the age of 40 may be worthwhile. Typically, the mammogram is repeated every 1 to 3 years. Ideally, it should pick up breast abnormalities prior to them becoming noticeable by the woman. Sometimes, lesions as small as 2–3mm can be picked up. At the other end of the spectrum, advanced cancers which spread to lymph nodes or other organs are becoming less common in screened populations of women as they are being detected and so the cancer can be treated in the early stage.

Mammography is well suited to the task of screening for many reasons. Most importantly, it will detect up to 85% of breast cancers in the age range described above. Second, it is a test that is very safe to administer, and whilst associated with some discomfort, is generally well tolerated by most women to the extent that they are happy to return at regular intervals for repeat screening. Mammography is also widely available and relatively cheap to perform. Government-backed programmes are generally provided as a free service to women in the appropriate age range.

Many women are concerned that breast implants may affect their ability to have a mammogram—in fact it is still safe and possible to have a mammogram with implants, but it is important that the woman lets the technician performing the test know as some special views may be required.

Detection of early breast cancers would be of no use if we were unable to then offer better treatment compared with that for more advanced cancers.

Mammogram screening programmes have, in fact, been shown to improve survival rates from breast cancer by up to 30%. Women whose cancers are detected by screening mammography also tend to have smaller tumours, and are therefore more likely to be able to have a lumpectomy rather than mastectomy.

> Screening programmes are well suited to detect breast cancer as
> they can detect disease early allowing more options for treatment
> and a better chance of cure.

The downside of screening

Unfortunately, there are some problems associated with any disease-screening
programme and specifically with mammography screening. At the most basic
level, there is an obvious inconvenience to women and the anxiety and discomfort of a mammogram. In addition, more than 1 in 100 screening mammograms
will lead to further testing which ultimately turns out to be negative for cancer.
More X-rays, ultrasound and MRI scans, needle biopsies and, occasionally, even
surgical biopsy under anaesthetic may be required which can lead to greater
anxiety and stress due to the fear of a cancer diagnosis.

Whilst testing may be ultimately negative for cancer, there are obvious costs to
the woman in terms of time, emotion and sometimes, discomfort. Needle and
surgical biopsies also carry a small risk of adverse consequences. Potentially
hundreds of women undergo negative testing for each woman who is diagnosed with cancer. The level of testing we as a community are willing to accept
with the aim of saving lives from breast cancer is ultimately a philosophical
question.

Table 4.1 Potentially negative aspects of screening

Anxiety, excess worry	About what might be found by a mammogram is normal
	Ask to have the mammography process explained to you
	Ask when you can expect to receive the results
Discomfort	Usually minimal during a mammogram
	Technique of the mammographer can help
	Local anaesthetic will be given before most biopsies
Further diagnostic tests	These may turn out to be unnecessary if the results are negative
	Costs to the woman in terms of time, emotional stress and possible discomfort
	Some tests have a small risk of adverse consequences
	These can be important to rule out suspicious lesions

There is also the issue of borderline breast lesions. This means lesions that are
not actual invasive cancers, may be precancerous or indicate in some other way
a cancer nearby. In the era before screening, the majority of these lesions would
simply not have been known about. Perhaps they became a problem, perhaps

they did not. Now that we are detecting these lesions so early, we are left with the problem of what to do about them. Our tendency has been to remove most given that we know there is at least some significant risk of associated cancer, but the doubt remains as to whether we are subjecting women to unnecessary tests and surgery due to breast screening.

Breast screening can also wrongly reassure women that everything is fine. It is well recognized that some women having their breast screen mammography already have a concern about their breasts—whether it be a lump they have noticed or some other symptom. Breast screening is not really set up to deal with this situation.

> **Any symptom should be fully assessed by a medical practitioner even in the event that the screening mammogram is all clear.**

A doctor can provide a more focused evaluation of a symptom as opposed to routine screening. A mammogram is just one way of looking at the breasts but will only detect around 80% of cancers, so any breast symptom should be reported to a doctor despite a clear mammogram.

Many women express concern about the radiation effects of repeated mammography. This is a reasonable concern as it is impossible to deny that radiation from X-rays can cause cancer. In reality though, the risk of this is minute; the chance of a mammogram causing breast cancer is less than 1 in a million. Even with repeated mammography over a lifetime, the risk remains incredibly small. For example, it is much more risky to use a car for a year.

New digital technology is making mammograms more accurate and means less radiation is needed.

Financial considerations

It is worth finally mentioning the cost of a breast-screening programme. Whilst it is usual that there is no cost to individual women, obviously, taxpayers foot the bill and have every reason to expect that their money is well spent. Whilst it would be nice to have unlimited financial means for combating disease, the reality is that the health budget of governments is not bottomless and so programmes such as breast screening must be able to provide good benefits in a cost-effective way. Various countries have analysed this in detail and have concluded that government-funded breast screening provides an excellent use of the health budget: in fact it saves lives in the long term, and also saves money given the financial cost to the community of cancer deaths.

📄 Case study

Valda is a nurse who works in health promotion in a small country town in rural Australia. The national breast screening programme has a van which visits the town every 2 years to offer free mammograms to all local women over 50. This van is equipped with a mammogram machine and a very experienced radiographer (X-ray technician) who can take the mammograms. The pictures are then sent to the city to be interpreted and women and their GPs are informed of the results within a few weeks.

Traditionally about half of women eligible for the screen would attend for a mammogram in the week the van is in town – this is quite a low participation rate and means the screening programme is less effective than it should be.

Valda has the task of coordinating the screening van visit. She advertises it widely not only in GP surgeries but via the local community centres, country women's organisations and at a local county fete where she has an information booth. Valda is also able to promote other health issues important to middle-aged and older women – it is winter and women are able to access flu vaccines, get advice about a local programme to get fit and loose weight, and join an aqua-aerobics programme at the new indoor swimming pool.

The community newspaper runs a series of health articles for Valda, and the local GPs get on board encouraging their patients to go for screening. The arrival of the screening van in town is a bit of an event – and local participation over the week rises to 75% of eligible women.

Some months on, at a de-briefing session by the breast screening programme Valda learns that of the 200 or so women screened that week, 2 were found to have cancer, and both of these were at a very early stage and likely to be completely cured by treatment.

5

Diagnosis of breast disease

> ## ➡ Key Points
>
> ◆ Eight out of ten breast symptoms are due to benign disease, NOT cancer.
> ◆ Breast symptoms usually need investigations including examination by a doctor, imaging (mammogram and/or ultrasound) and a needle biopsy.
> ◆ If cancer is diagnosed the type of cancer (pathology) will determine the outlook.

Breast symptoms are common, and most are found to be due not to cancer but to a range of benign changes from the normal hormonal changes of the breast tissue to benign lumps such as fibroadenomas or even chronic infective conditions. However, all new breast changes that persist for some weeks should be investigated and this chapter outlines the possible tests that may be done, and thus how a diagnosis of the breast change is made.

Diagnosis

Although some breast cancers are picked up by a screening mammogram (Chapter 4) most cancers are found after the woman herself (or sometimes her partner) finds a breast change. Sometimes a breast cancer is detected when a doctor such as the woman's GP does a routine breast check.

Any new breast symptom which is not obviously hormonal breast change (and thus resolves during the course of the menstrual cycle) should be investigated with a triple test. This means a clinical examination, some kind of imaging and a biopsy. These are described below.

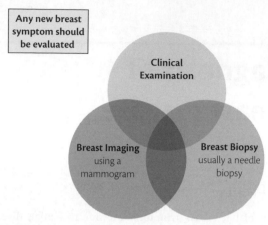

Any new breast symptom should be evaluated

Clinical Examination

Breast Imaging
using a
mammogram

Breast Biopsy
usually a needle
biopsy

Figure 5.1 The triple test.

Clinical examination

The examination of a woman's breast by a doctor is much like that described in Chapter 3 on self-examination—looking for changes in the shape, colour or size of the breast and nipple and feeling the breast and under the arm for any lumps or other abnormalities. Tenderness is usually associated with hormonal breast change but can rarely be a sign of cancer.

If a woman presents to her GP with a breast symptom she may be referred directly to the appropriate specialist, such as a radiologist for the tests outlined below, or directly to a specialist breast clinic who will arrange all the tests, often on one day.

Breast tests—imaging
Mammogram

This is another way of describing a breast X-ray. Mammography is the commonest test used to diagnose a breast problem, although it is of most use in women over 40, as younger women have very dense breast tissue which makes reading the mammogram difficult in some cases. However, if the doctor is concerned a breast symptom may be cancer, a mammogram should be performed regardless of the woman's age.

Mammograms do not detect all breast cancers—even in older women with breast tissue that is easy to X-ray, less than 90% of cancers are seen on a mammogram.

During the mammogram the breast is placed between metallic plates which compress the breast tissue. Two or three different angles may be taken and in some situations, focused views of particular areas of concern may be requested. The X-ray pictures can be developed almost instantly, although reading them can take a little more time and is best done by two radiologists trained in breast imaging. The radiation dose from a mammogram is extremely small and equivalent to less than a year of normal background radiation from our environment.

Benign lumps are typically rounded and smooth-edged. Cancers, by contrast, may be denser in the middle with an irregular edge. The surrounding breast tissue may be distorted by the cancerous invasion. Sometimes, cancerous change may be associated with clusters of calcium flecks which show up on a mammogram as bright white dots (calcification).

Ultrasound

Ultrasound uses sound waves to create a picture of the breast tissue and distinguish different structures. Many women are familiar with ultrasound from pregnancy—many parents' first picture of their child is an ultrasound one! Because it does not use radiation it is a harmless test and also painless. However, ultrasound is very dependent on the experience of the person performing it, and is also not a good way to 'screen' a whole breast, but is an excellent way to look closely at a particular area of concern, particularly if that area needs to be 'targeted' for a biopsy.

Like mammograms, breast ultrasounds do not detect all cancers, but in combination with a mammogram are extremely accurate—over 95% of cancers will be seen.

Because breast density does not affect the ability of the doctor to read them, they are as useful in women of all ages.

Magnetic resonance imaging

Breast magnetic resonance imaging (MRI) is a very complex imaging test which is done for screening young women at very high risk of breast cancer (see Chapter 2) and occasionally in women with suspected breast cancer but where other tests cannot prove the diagnosis. It is also sometimes done in women with known cancer to measure the size of the tumour or its response to treatments, or to look for subtle changes which may indicate recurrence. It is a test which takes a lot of expertise to interpret, and so can only be done by relatively few experienced radiologists, and should be ordered by a specialist team in conjunction with other tests and examination. It may also have a significant cost involved as it is not always covered by government payments or insurance.

An MRI uses a very high magnetic field to create small electrical currents which are then converted into images which are highly accurate in distinguishing different tissues from each other depending on factors such as their blood supply—in particular cancer. Usually an injected contrast agent (a kind of dye) is used, called gadolinium, which highlights these changes on the images.

For a woman, the MRI will mean lying for up to 40 minutes in a long tube with the breast placed in cups under the body. It may be quite noisy and some women may find it claustrophobic.

Breast test—biopsies

Fine-needle aspiration

Fine-needle aspiration (FNA) means collecting a small sample of cells from an area of change such as a lump in the breast using a very thin needle and syringe. It is done either by a pathologist or in a specialist breast clinic. It may also be done using ultrasound or a mammogram to direct the needle (often by a radiologist), especially if the area of concern is not felt but only seen on imaging.

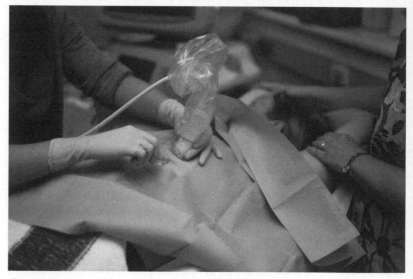

Figure 5.2 Ultrasound-guided fine needle aspiration.

The procedure can be done using some local anaesthetic to numb the breast first.

Once the cells have been aspirated (or sucked out) they are given to a pathologist to stain and interpret—this is a highly technical task, and can take a day or so, although many clinics are able to offer a 'one-stop' service where the FNA is read in the clinic within an hour or so. Unfortunately this test is not always able to give the patient and doctor a definitive answer and further biopsies may be needed.

Core/mammotome biopsy

Like FNA, core biopsy (mammotome is just the name for a different kind of needle) uses a needle to remove some breast—only this time one or more small 'worms' of tissue rather than just a few cells. Again the procedure can be done directly on a palpable lump or using imaging guidance. Local anaesthetic is used and a tiny nick is made in the skin prior the needle being inserted. This does not require a stitch however and heals up with virtually no scar.

The tissue from a core biopsy needs special processing which usually takes a few days, although some clinics offer imprint cytology which means essentially getting a few cells from the core of tissue and processing these in an hour or so which may (but not always) give a result. The advantage of core biopsy over FNA is that is gives more tissue for the pathologist to work on, and thus may be both more accurate and allow a larger range of tests to be done, particularly if the lump is a cancer.

Open surgical biopsy

Fortunately very few women have to have an operation to diagnose their breast problem, as the techniques above will be able to distinguish benign problems from cancer in the vast majority of cases. This is especially true if a woman presents with a breast lump. However, breast screening programmes often find changes which are extremely difficult to diagnose, or which may be benign in themselves but occasionally associated with cancer. In this instance a woman may be advised to have the area of concern removed with an operation. As these areas are often not palpable this may mean localizing the area prior to surgery—this is done by placing a fine wire into the lesion using ultrasound or a mammogram machine (done on the morning of the operation) so the surgeon can locate the exact area to remove at operation (see Chapter 8).

A diagnostic open surgical biopsy aims to remove only a small volume of tissue, so although the woman requires an operation and general anaesthetic (usually as a day case procedure), scarring and distortion should be minimal.

Diagnosis of the spread of cancer

The vast majority of women with early breast cancer will have it localized to the breast plus or minus some lymph glands under the arm. Thus for most women there is no benefit in even looking elsewhere in the body for spread. However, for women with larger or more aggressive cancers, the specialists may recommend tests to exclude spread to elsewhere: these are called metastases and are discussed further in Chapter 13. These will usually include blood tests (a full blood count and liver function tests and calcium levels which can rise if cancer reaches the bones), imaging of the liver and lungs (by either chest X-ray and ultrasound or CT scan) and a bone scan. All of these tests are very straightforward and easy to tolerate.

📄 Case study

Maria is a 38-year-old woman recently immigrated from Southern Europe who noticed a breast lump on the left side in the upper outer part of the breast. She needed to find a GP, and by the time she did so and reported the lump, which took about two months, the GP estimated it was 2cm in size, but very smooth and felt like a cyst. The GP requested an ultrasound and this was reported as a cyst, so Maria was reassured and told no further treatment was needed.

She continued to feel the lump over the next four months and felt it may be getting bigger. Although her GP has explained that it was important to return if it did increase in size she had not really understood this, and was worried about 'bothering' the doctor again. However eventually her 17 year old daughter persuaded her it was important to go again to the GP and this time the lump was 5 cm in size.

Maria was referred to the local breast clinic where a mammogram, ultrasound and core biopsy were done which showed a fairly large breast cancer.

6

Breast cancer under the microscope

How pathology relates to the course of the disease

> ## ⮕ Key Points
>
> ◆ A pathologist will look at a sample of tumour cells under a microscope to diagnose the type of breast cancer.
>
> ◆ Staging of the tumour is determined by several factors including grade, lymph node involvement, size and responsiveness to hormones.
>
> ◆ Prognosis can inform the patient of the likelihood that treatment will be able to eradicate cancer and prevent it ever recurring in the future.

This chapter discusses what types of breast cancer there are, how features of an individual cancer relate to how it will behave and how likely it is to recur after treatment or even prove fatal.

What is breast cancer?

Cancer is a term which covers an incredibly diverse range of conditions that can potentially affect any part of the human body. The characteristic feature of all cancers is that the usual balance between cell multiplication and cell death is lost. Whilst cells all over our bodies are damaged regularly, our immune system will usually either repair or destroy them. If for some reason a cell becomes resistant to these control mechanisms, it may start multiplying out of control—a tumour is born. It is not likely to be one error within the cells which leads to a tumour but more commonly a series of failures which leads to the problem.

> So breast cancer is a disease that occurs when the natural checks and balances that keep our cells under control—regularly developing, dividing, dying off and functioning normally—somehow go awry.

In breast cancer the cells affected are either those lining the breast ducts which transfer milk during breastfeeding (ductal cancer) or the lobules where milk is made (lobular cancer). The degree to which the cancer cells have altered from how a normal cell looks and functions is related to how aggressively the cancer behaves—this is the tumour grade.

Because it has the ability to keep dividing into new cells and loses the normal ability to die off when old and not working well, a cancer cell loses some of the normal behaviour of a breast cell called programmed cell death. A cancer cell also gains the ability to move both within the breast and via blood vessels and lymphatic vessels to other areas of the body where it may continue to divide and grow.

The reasons a cancer develops are extremely complex and even now they are not completely understood. Every cell contains a genetic code which dictates how it functions—whether it is a breast cell, a nerve cell or a cardiac muscle cell—but in cancer a series of genes get turned on or off when they are not supposed to, making the cell function abnormally and a cancer develops. This leads the cancer cells to display the typical behaviour of a cancer—they can grow, multiply and spread almost unchecked. The details of these changes are what is called the pathological features of the tumour.

The pathology of breast cancer

Pathology is the study of tissues under the microscope, which allows us to make a diagnosis of a disease.

Type of cancer

Breast cancer can arise in ducts or lobules—ductal and lobular cancer. There are some other rarer types of cancer, and their names usually reflect what the cells look like to the pathologist under the microscope.

Another fundamental feature of breast cancer is that some are *in situ* (or in one place) and some invasive. *In-situ* breast cancer (usually of the duct cells—ductal carcinoma *in situ* or DCIS) is a condition which usually is found when changes are seen on a mammogram—generally as calcification or tiny white dots of calcium which are laid down in the ducts as the condition develops. In DCIS the cells lining the breast ducts undergo some of the changes of breast cancer: they keep dividing and certainly look abnormal under the microscope, but do not yet have the ability to spread anywhere else in the body. Thus DCIS is a disease confined to the breast and can be cured by removing all of the area affected (often with radiotherapy as well). If not treated at this stage a large proportion of DCIS will go on to become actual breast cancer, with the ability to spread, and so threaten life.

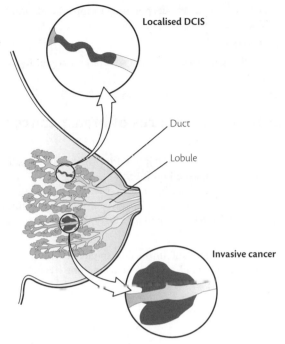

Localised DCIS

Duct

Lobule

Invasive cancer

Figure 6.1 Ductal carcinoma *in situ.*

There is also a condition called LCIS or lobular carcinoma *in situ.* This again rarely presents as a lump and in fact is virtually always a chance finding on breast biopsy. LCIS is rarely a precursor of cancer, but does signify a woman is at considerably higher risk than normal of developing a breast cancer in the future—perhaps up to five times more—and this risk is of breast cancer on either side.

Besides actual cancer there are a whole group of conditions which are sometimes identified when a woman has a breast biopsy—these are benign but signify an increase in risk of future breast cancer. These include atypical ductal hyperplasia (ADH) and atypical lobular hyperplasia (ALH).

It is important to note that most women with these changes will not develop breast cancer, but are usually advised to undergo more frequent screening mammograms, for example each year, so if a breast cancer does develop there is the best chance of detecting it very early.

Cancer grade

The grade of a cancer represents how aggressive the cancer cells look under the microscope and how different they are from a normal breast cell. This is correlated to the aggressiveness of the cancer—its potential to spread and ultimately threaten a woman's life. There are three grades of cancer:

Grade 1: least aggressive

Grade 2: moderately aggressive (lobular cancers and some ductal cancers are usually this grade)

Grade 3: most likely to grow quickly and spread.

Other pathological features of breast cancer
Lymph node involvement

Perhaps the most important factor to know for prognosis is whether the cancer has spread to lymph nodes, usually under the arm (the axilla). If a patient has enlarged lymph nodes, these can be biopsied with a needle prior to surgery. If they are involved the woman is usually advised to undergo surgical removal of most of these lymph nodes—an axillary clearance—both to treat this and to ascertain how many are involved.

If no lymph nodes are felt it is still important to check that there are no microscopic deposits of cancer spread to them. This is done by axillary clearance or sentinel node biopsy (Chapter 8).

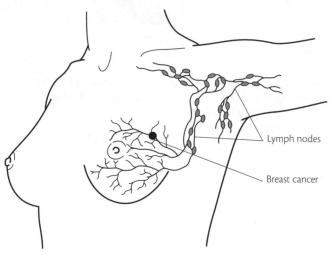

Figure 6.2 Lymph nodes.

The presence of tumour in lymph nodes and the number of involved nodes is directly related to the aggressiveness of the cancer.

Most women with involved lymph nodes will be offered systemic treatment, such as chemotherapy (Chapter 10).

Tumour size and lympho-vascular invasion

The size of a tumour is also important in estimating how aggressive a cancer is and predicting the outcome of the disease—certainly tumours less than 2cm usually have a very good outlook.

A pathologist will report on whether the tiny vessels immediately around the tumour have cancer cells in them—called lympho-vascular invasion (LVI). This indicates the cancer has a higher chance of coming back locally and so the surgeon and radiotherapist may advocate more radical local treatment.

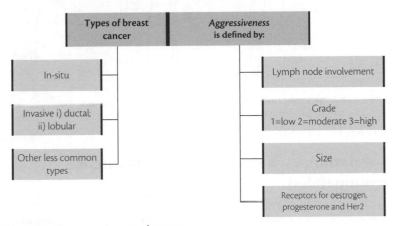

Figure 6.3 The aggressiveness of cancer.

Receptors

Other important tests done on the removed tumour by the pathologist are testing for hormone receptors—oestrogen receptors (ER) and progesterone receptors (PgR)—as well as looking for the growth factor receptor called Her2 (or cerbB2).

These receptors are important in predicting the aggressiveness of a cancer. ER and PgR positive cancers are often *less* aggressive whilst Her2 positive cancers are *more* aggressive. Receptors also guide which treatments will work. Women whose tumours are ER and/or PgR positive can have hormone treatments (such as Tamoxifen) to decrease the chance of recurrence and improve survival (Chapter 11), whilst women whose tumours are Her2 positive can have the drug Trastuzumab (better known as Herceptin—see Chapter 12).

Putting these features together is called 'staging' the cancer. Most of this information comes from the pathologist after the breast cancer has been removed, although some can come from a needle biopsy and from other tests which look for spread of cancer to other organs.

Taking all of these pathology staging factors together, the treating doctors can give a patient an estimate of her prognosis—or how likely treatment will be able to eradicate cancer and prevent it ever recurring in the future. Some of the pathology features will also guide which treatments are recommended.

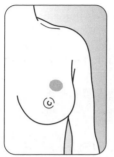 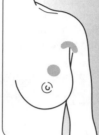 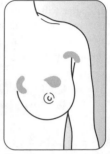

Stage 1:
Early disease tumour confined to the breast

Stage 2:
Early disease

Stage 3:
Local advanced disease tumour

Figure 6.4 Tumour stages.

How pathology is related to the treatment recommended

The following box shows a general view of why doctors may recommend different treatments. Again each decision is individual, and not only the cancer factors are important, but the woman's viewpoint and her general health.

Pathological features guiding treatment recommendations

- ER/PgR positive: hormone treatments usually recommended
- Moderate or poor-risk tumours: chemotherapy usually recommended
- ER/PgR negative: chemotherapy usually recommended, especially in younger women
- Her2 (cerbB2) positive: Herceptin usually recommended

Question to ask the doctor: What kind of breast cancer do I have?

This means the type of cancer, the grade, if it has spread to lymph glands and what receptors are positive.

How pathology is related to the course of the cancer

Breast cancers can be divided into tumours of different potential prognosis depending on the factors described above (their potential aggressiveness). The box shows average figures for prognosis—no one can predict exactly how an individual woman will respond to treatment and if her cancer will recur.

> **A woman's general health is also important to her outcome.**

Distant staging

Women with poor prognosis cancers have a higher likelihood that the disease will spread elsewhere, so these women will often be recommended to have tests to check this. The most likely sites of spread are to bone, lungs and liver, so these tests will usually include blood tests, a bone scan and CT scans, or a chest X-ray and ultrasound of the liver. It is important to remember these tests can only pick up disease when it is more than a centimetre in size—microscopic deposits of cancer cannot been seen.

> **Question to ask your doctor: Should I have tests of the rest of my body for cancer?**
>
> *This is most useful if the cancer is more aggressive or has spread to lymph nodes.*

Advances in pathology

In terms of predicting the outcome for an individual patient of whether her tumour may return, one of the most exciting current developments is the advent of 'molecular fingerprinting' (or microarray technology) which looks at a large number of genes in the tumour. This may predict both the aggressiveness of the cancer and how it may respond to treatments such as chemotherapy, but it is still in its infancy and much research is needed until it can reliably be used in routine practice.

How long has the cancer been present?

This is a common question a woman and her family ask, and for an individual is almost impossible to say. However, we know the 'average' breast cancer cell doubles every 100 days, and so until it reaches 1cm in size (or a million cells) and can first be felt and seen on a mammogram, it is likely to have been present quite a number of years.

> **Question to ask your doctor: What chance does my breast cancer have of returning?**
>
> *This will depend on the pathological features of the tumour, and the treatment received.*

Table 6.1 Pathology

Prognosis	Pathological feature				Treatment			
	Oestrogen status	Progesterone status	Size	LN spread	Surgery	RXT	Hormone therapy	Chemotherapy
Good	+	+	Less than 2cm	No	✓	✓	✓	✗
Moderate	+	+	More than 2cm	A few	✓	✓	✓	✓ (especially if less than 60 years old)
Poor	–	–	More than 5cm	Yes	✓	✓	Herceptin if Her2 + ✓ if ER/ PgR +	✓

LN, lymph node; RXT, radiotherapy.

7

The team approach

> **➲ Key Points**
>
> ◆ Multidisciplinary care, provided by a team of medical professionals, is the current approach to manage breast cancer.
>
> ◆ The multidisciplinary team consists of a range of professionals including a:
>
> General practitioner
>
> Radiologist
>
> Breast surgeon and sometimes plastic surgeon
>
> Specialist breast nurse
>
> Medical oncologist
>
> Radiation oncologist
>
> Physiotherapist and occupational therapist
>
> Psychologist
>
> Social worker
>
> Researcher
>
> Patient
>
> ◆ The combined expertise of a multidisciplinary team will be used to help formulate the most appropriate treatment plan for the patient.

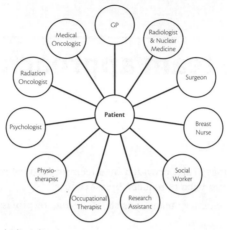

Figure 7.1 The multidisciplinary team.

The term 'journey' is used by many women in the context of their breast cancer diagnosis and treatment. It is an appropriate term to describe what can be a long process involving lots of tests, advice and treatment. Some women are surprised at just how many people are involved in their care—from general practitioner to breast surgeon and nurse, to the oncology team and so on. This is the basis of modern management of breast cancer. It is not the domain of an individual doctor to take sole responsibility for a patient. Rather, given the complexities involved in the diagnosis and treatment of breast cancer, it has been conclusively shown that women benefit from multidisciplinary care. This is another way of describing a treating team who utilize their wide range of individual skills to care for the patient and her family.

General practitioner

Often it is the GP who will first pick up breast change and investigate a lump or other symptom reported by a patient. GPs are well positioned to support a woman through potentially months of treatment and to monitor her once the acute treatment period is over.

Whilst most women will not have met other members of the treating team before, their GPs can be a constant and trusted coordinator through the whole process. GPs are also an invaluable means by which to reinforce information from other sources which may only have been partially understood previously. In rural areas, where easy access to the full range of health services can be limited, GPs commonly shoulder more of the load in a shared care treatment plan between them and other health practitioners.

Radiologists and breast screening

An increasing number of breast lesions which cannot be felt are being detected through the use of screening tests such as mammography. This may be within a formal government-sponsored breast screening programme, operating independently from GP visits or, alternatively, through clinics after referral from a GP.

Radiologists are doctors who interpret X-rays and other scans. They are integral in breast cancer care due to the heavy reliance placed on mammograms, ultrasound, CT, MRI and other imaging techniques. Once a concerning lesion has been found, further assessment is driven by these doctors, in consultation with other members of the multidisciplinary team, until a diagnosis is made—often by radiologically guided needle biopsy. Radiologists may also have a role to play in helping surgeons remove breast lesions which are too small to feel, and finally, are critical in monitoring women after breast cancer—both to watch for cancer relapse as well as new cancers.

Surgeons

Breast surgeons are general surgeons with added expertise in assessing and treating breast disease. They can help in diagnosing a breast problem when the GP is not sure of the best way to proceed. Alternatively, they may just get involved when a diagnosis has already been made by the GP and/or breast screening service. Regardless, breast surgeons will often organize further testing in order to optimize any treatment plan. Treatments differ depending on the type of cancer and how advanced it is, as well as patient characteristics such as other medical problems, age and treatment preference. Sometimes, if the surgeon feels that surgery is not the best option, he or she may refer a woman with newly diagnosed breast cancer on to another specialist such as a medical or radiation oncologist.

> Surgery is usually the first step in treatment which is why surgeons do tend to coordinate this initial period.

When necessary, the breast surgeon will involve a plastic surgeon to help with cosmetic issues after mastectomy and occasionally, lumpectomy. The two surgeons may work together in removing the cancer and reconstructing the breast or the plastic surgeon may come into the picture later on.

Breast surgeons will often be involved in non-surgical aspects of patient care too. Hormonal therapy and managing side-effects of treatment are examples of this. After cancer, a woman will need to be watched closely for relapse or new cancers. This is usually done by a combination of the doctors involved and may involve visits to the surgeon. It is very useful for surgeons to remain thus involved as they have often been involved with the patient from early on in her treatment course and have a good feel for what has transpired. In addition, some women will require more surgery, should they develop more disease.

Breast nurses

Breast nurses are trained to help with the specific issues facing breast cancer sufferers. They commonly work with breast surgeons and therefore are involved early on in the breast cancer journey. Doctors have been criticised for not treating a patient 'holistically', but rather being too disease-focused. Breast nurses can fill some of this treatment void by overseeing the entire process and, through their experience and training, pre-empt and address common problems. Women are often lost in a flurry of instruction and information after medical consults but may be too anxious or apprehensive to question the 'busy doctor'.

Breast nurses provide an easy-to-access and sometimes less confronting person to seek help from. As with other members of the multidisciplinary treating team, they bring an area of expertise to cancer care that may make treatment and its aftermath easier to get through. Problems with bras and/or prostheses after surgery, the hormonal effects of treatment, relationship and economic stresses that a cancer diagnosis may precipitate are all areas that women often feel more comfortable discussing with their nurse rather than doctor.

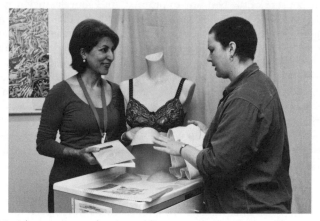

Figure 7.2 A breast nurse and patient with mannequin, prosthesis and bra.

Breast nurses are uniquely placed within the hospital or breast clinic to provide a constant point of reference for women throughout their treatment.

Medical oncologist

Medical oncology relates to drug rather than surgical treatment of cancer. It most commonly involves chemotherapy, but medical oncologists do much more than just administer chemotherapy. Their involvement in breast cancer may start at diagnosis in planning the best course of treatment when surgery is not ideal. More commonly, after surgery, if there is a significant risk of cancer deposits still in the body, they will be involved in planning some form of treatment to try and kill off these cells.

The medical oncologist coordinates drug treatments in early and advanced breast cancer. As well or instead of chemotherapy, they may recommend hormonal therapy or other, newer forms of treatment (Chapters 10, 11 and 12). Their role also encompasses looking after any side-effects of these treatments, which can be quite serious. Finally, medical oncologists may share in the long-term monitoring of women after breast cancer and are very prominent in treating cancer recurrence.

Radiation oncologist

Many women with breast cancer will require radiotherapy at some point. Radiation oncologists plan and administer radiotherapy as well as monitor the outcome, both in terms of cancer control and side-effects.

It is important for the radiation oncologist to be involved early on, in order to recommend which women should receive radiation to optimize their cancer treatment. Radiotherapy is usually given after surgery and any chemotherapy needed, although planning for it may start as soon as it is known that it is required. Radiotherapy may also be used later on for cancer relapse. It is discussed in detail in Chapter 9.

Physiotherapist

Breast cancer treatment, surgery in particular, can lead to problems such as shoulder stiffness and lymphoedema of the arm or breast. Regular exercises as well as physical therapy instigated by a physiotherapist may be extremely beneficial in preventing or treating these problems.

Women would benefit from seeing a physiotherapist both before and after surgery as well as at any other time that problems develop. In addition, some centres run classes to further reinforce what women can do to improve their outcomes after treatment. This is discussed in Chapter 16.

Occupational therapist

In some centres, occupational therapists may perform a role similar to that of the physiotherapist. They are also often involved in the prevention and management of lymphoedema through the use of elastic compression sleeves for the arm in question. Whilst these sleeves can be bought in standard sizes, occupational therapists are able to construct specially shaped ones for more challenging situations where the standard sleeve is not achieving maximum benefit.

Psychologist

Some women will deal with the psychological impact of a cancer diagnosis and its treatment more easily than others. At the very least, there is an inevitable feeling of grief and fear, for the woman involved as well as family members. Psychologists are commonly employed to talk through these issues and instigate further treatment as required. They may help a woman understand her feelings better in ultimately coming to the right decisions for her in her treatment, thus facilitating the best outcome, as discussed in Chapter 14. It is best to start this process early on when it is evident that a woman is not coping as well as she could.

Social worker

It is important to recognize that cancer creates social stress for many people. Treatment may involve time off work and/or away from family and friends as well as added costs. These social problems add to the already great strain that is present and can ultimately impact on treatment. Social assistance is available from many organizations—often the biggest problem is finding them.

A social worker is well placed to help women gain the support they may need to optimize their treatment. This will be further discussed in Chapter 14.

Research assistant

Research is a critical part of breast cancer care. Much of what we know and use today has come out of clinical research. There is a great deal of effort being put into breast cancer research in an attempt to continually improve treatment. A big part of this involves clinical trials where new treatments are assessed in patients (Chapter 12). Certainly, a lot of what we know today has come out of historical trials, which have tracked the experiences of hundreds of thousands of breast cancer sufferers. It is imperative that as many women as possible have access to ongoing trials so as to maximize our future knowledge. By entering trials now, patients can add to the body of knowledge available to better treat breast cancer in the future. In addition, they may gain access to new treatments that are otherwise not available to them. Facilitating all of this are the researchers who are employed or volunteer to coordinate trial participation. It would not be possible to run large, effective trials without them.

'The rest'

There are many others involved in looking after women with breast cancer and their families. These include administrative staff, radiographers, anaesthetists and often other specialists. Many clinics also contain volunteers to further enhance the service. It truly is a multidisciplinary model of health care, which has revolutionized the way in which patients are treated. Much of the experience from multidisciplinary care of breast cancer has been utilized to set up similar systems in other areas of disease.

Multidisciplinary meetings

A big part of effective multidisciplinary care revolves around excellent communication and coordination between those involved. The easiest way to do this is by regular meetings where patients are discussed and a treatment plan made. This is the easiest way to bring the combined expertise of the multidisciplinary team into action. Patients with complex problems may be discussed at multiple meetings as information comes to hand. Such an approach gives comfort to both patients and the treating team alike, knowing that any decisions made have been thoroughly considered from all angles to provide the best care available.

8

Surgery for breast cancer

➜ Key Points

◆ Surgery is usually the first treatment for breast cancer.

◆ Surgical options for the breast include mastectomy and breast-conserving surgery.

◆ Some kind of axillary surgery is needed for most women with invasive breast cancer.

Surgery is the first step in the treatment pathway for most women with breast cancer. Traditionally, this has meant excision of all breast tissue from the affected side (mastectomy) as well as the lymph glands from under that arm (axillary clearance). Advances in our understanding of breast cancer and its treatment over the past 20 years have meant that many women are able to be offered less extensive surgery, without reducing the overall cure rate. Cure of the cancer is the main goal, but how the scars will look, access to radiotherapy services and concerns about future cancers are also important when deciding on what surgery to conduct.

> **Two women with identical cancers may have quite different surgery with no difference in their subsequent chance of cure.**

Options that may be discussed include mastectomy or double mastectomy—with or without breast reconstruction—versus breast-conserving therapy, and complete removal of axillary lymph glands versus diagnostic sampling of the lymph glands.

> **Question to ask the doctor: Will you know if you haven't got all of the cancer out?**
>
> *Once the cancer is removed at surgery, it is sent to the pathology laboratory for analysis. Part of this involves assessing the specimen to ensure that the cancer is surrounded by healthy tissue on all sides meaning that none has been inadvertently left behind. It takes a few days to get the full pathology testing done so when necessary, further excision is done at a second operation.*

Breast-conserving surgery

Wide local excision or lumpectomy of a breast cancer means removal of the cancer itself as well as a cuff, or margin, of surrounding normal tissue—usually about 10mm worth. Patients often think of this as a 'lumpectomy' although strictly speaking, lumpectomy refers to the excision of any breast lump without necessarily a margin of normal breast tissue around it. Wide local excision is ideal for smaller cancers if a good cosmetic result for the remainder of the breast can be achieved.

Wide local excision may be a good option for some larger cancers if their location within the breast and the breast's overall size allows a good cosmetic result. Larger cancers can sometimes be shrunk with chemotherapy, so enabling breast-conserving surgery (Chapter 10).

Breast-conserving surgery, if possible, is preferable for many women as it may allow them to cope better, maintain better self-image and quality of life.

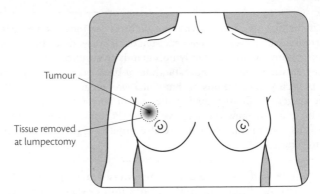

Figure 8.1 A woman with a lumpectomy.

There are downsides to breast-conserving surgery, however. Preoperative X-rays, scans and biopsy may underestimate the amount of cancer or precancerous (preinvasive) tissue in the breast. Attempted wide local excision of the cancer may fail to achieve adequate cancer clearance. In fact, about 20% of women require a second operation. Mastectomy may even be the end result if disease in the breast turns out to be much more widespread than anticipated.

> After breast-conserving surgery almost all women will need radiotherapy to the remaining breast tissue on the affected side to minimise the risk of cancer returning in that breast.

Radiotherapy is discussed in the next chapter.

Wide local excision of a breast cancer along with radiotherapy is known as breast-conserving therapy and has an equivalent long-term cure rate to mastectomy for any given patient. Without subsequent radiotherapy, the risk of cancer returning in the remaining breast tissue is very high—up to 30%.

Finally, despite careful preoperative planning, the cosmetic result after breast-conserving surgery may occasionally fall short of what is acceptable to the patient. This can mean revisional surgery or even conversion to mastectomy with or without breast reconstruction.

Hookwire localization of breast cancer

Many small breast cancers are very difficult or impossible to feel. These cancers are known as impalpable and are usually detected via screening mammograms. Whilst finding them so small usually means the disease has been caught at an early stage, it does bring added complexity to the operation. If a woman has chosen to have a mastectomy, then it is not important to be able to feel the cancer in the breast as the whole breast is being removed anyway. However, in breast-conserving surgery, the surgeon needs to accurately work out which part of the breast to remove and so uses the technique of hookwire localized wide local excision.

On the day prior or morning of the operation, a sterilized wire, about as thin as an injection needle, is placed into the breast using X-ray or ultrasound guidance. The idea is to get the tip of the wire close to or into the lesion being removed. This is known as hookwire localization and is usually done by a radiologist. The patient is awake, but a local anaesthetic injection is used so as to minimize any pain. The surgeon is able to use the wire as a guide to remove the cancer. This specimen is then X-rayed to ensure that the cancer is all removed.

A second operation is sometimes needed if the final pathology suggests there may be some tumour left in the breast.

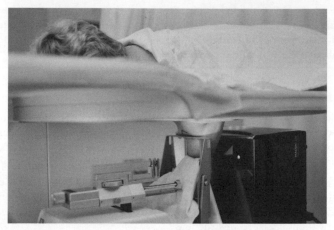

Figure 8.2 A hookwire localization.

> **Question to ask the doctor: Will I wake up with a mastectomy if you feel you can't save the breast?**
>
> *Your doctor will never proceed to performing a mastectomy if he or she has not discussed it with you beforehand.*

Mastectomy

Mastectomy relates to removal of all breast tissue and is a good treatment option for many women. Alternatively, if there is extensive precancerous disease in the breast, a surgeon may be unhappy to avoid mastectomy given the very real chance of a second cancer lat er in life. Some women who have breast cancer across many family members may find development of their own cancer a compelling reason to undergo mastectomy, or even double mastectomy, in an effort to minimize their risk of subsequent cancers. This is particularly relevant when there is a known breast cancer gene within the family (see Chapter 2). Finally, for most women, mastectomy for breast cancer will do away with the need for radiotherapy. This in itself may be a reason to opt for mastectomy.

> **Mastectomy is most commonly recommended when breast conservation surgery is not possible due to the size of the tumour in relation to the size of the breast or when cancer is not confined to one spot within the breast.**

There are many types of mastectomy. Terms include simple mastectomy, skin-sparing or subcutaneous mastectomy, radical or modified radical mastectomy, prophylactic and bilateral mastectomy.

Simple mastectomy is an operation whereby all breast tissue as well as excess skin is removed from one side. After this excision, the skin is stitched together to leave a neat scar either horizontally or, more commonly, diagonally across one side of the chest where the breast was.

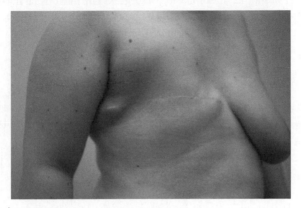

Figure 8.3 A mastectomy.

Skin-sparing and subcutaneous mastectomy are techniques in which breast tissue is removed, but not the overlying skin. The excess skin can be incorporated into a reconstructed breast. In a skin-sparing mastectomy, the nipple and areola are excised along with the breast tissue. Subcutaneous mastectomy is where the nipple and areola are kept.

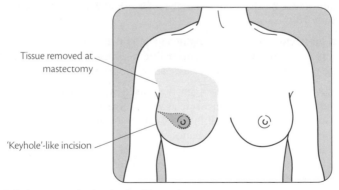

Tissue removed at mastectomy

'Keyhole'-like incision

Figure 8.4 A woman who has had a skin-sparing mastectomy.

Radical mastectomy is rarely done nowadays—it involves removal of the entire breast, axillary (under the arm) lymph glands and muscle from the chest underlying the breast. It is a disfiguring operation; even now, many women are upset at the thought of mastectomy having seen the poor cosmetic result in their grandmother or mother after this type of surgery. The most usual mastectomy is a modified radical mastectomy, in which chest muscle is not removed.

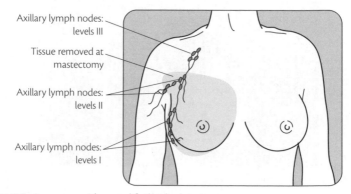

Axillary lymph nodes: levels III

Tissue removed at mastectomy

Axillary lymph nodes: levels II

Axillary lymph nodes: levels I

Figure 8.5 A woman with a modified radical mastectomy.

Prophylactic mastectomy refers to mastectomy undertaken when there is no cancer present in the breast. It is an appropriate choice for some women who are at particular risk of developing breast cancer and are keen to reduce that risk. Prophylactic mastectomy will reduce the risk of breast cancer on that side by virtually 100%.

Bilateral mastectomy means both right- and left-sided mastectomy. Occasionally, bilateral mastectomy may be undertaken due to a diagnosis of bilateral cancers, but more often it is performed, at least partly, for prophylactic reasons.

It is a common reaction in women diagnosed with cancer on one side to request mastectomy on the other side as well. Surgery on the unaffected breast will not improve the outcome of the known breast cancer. There may, however, be some benefit in reducing the chance of a second breast cancer in the future. Any woman who has had breast cancer is at an increased risk of a second breast cancer compared to the average population. The risk is up to 10% over the ensuing decade.

> **There is a high chance that a woman who has had one breast cancer will not develop another cancer.**

In addition, given the fact that she will be watched closely with regular mammograms, any new breast cancer is likely to be detected early, at a curable phase. There are a small group of women who are at high risk of developing breast cancer due to the likelihood of a breast cancer gene in their family (Chapter 2). These women may choose to undergo bilateral prophylactic mastectomy. Some women have lesions found on screening mammogram which, whilst not cancer, indicate a predisposition towards developing cancer. These women should be watched closely and sometimes prophylactic breast surgery may be an appropriate step.

The decision towards prophylactic mastectomy is not an easy one. It should be made only after careful consideration and discussion with the breast care team. Psychologists experienced in the breast area can be particularly useful in exploring the reasons a woman may be seeking this type of surgery as well as in dealing with some of the mental and emotional issues involved.

Axillary staging

Breast cancer can invade into the lymphatic channels and pass to the lymph glands where they may lodge and grow. Whether or not the lymph glands have been invaded by cancer is assessed by removing some or all of them and is called axillary staging. This can have important ramifications for a woman's treatment after her surgery. It is important to remove involved lymph glands as cancer relapse in them can be difficult to treat and may compromise the chance of cure.

As with the breast, surgery to the glands has become less extensive as our understanding of breast cancer has grown.

Axillary clearance

Axillary clearance is done if there is a suspicion of cancer being in the glands. It involves removal of the majority of lymph glands—usually about ten to twenty—from the armpit on the cancer side. The advantage of this approach is that it allows accurate staging of the axilla and removes any cancer there. If a mastectomy is being performed it is usually done through the same incision. If not, a separate cut under the arm is needed.

Removing these lymph glands can lead to lymphoedema. This occurs when tissue fluid in the arm or breast builds up (Chapter 16). Lymphoedema occurs in about 10–20% of patients after axillary clearance.

Shoulder stiffness is common after axillary surgery, but can usually be helped by exercise and physiotherapy. Sensory change in the skin of the upper inner arm is common (numbness or burning) and rarely damage to nerves leading to shoulder weakness.

This potential for complications has led to the development of sentinel lymph node biopsy. This is an alternate way by which to stage the axilla—determine whether there is cancer there—without the need to resort to a full axillary clearance in the absence of cancerous spread.

Sentinel lymph node biopsy

The term 'sentinel' means guard. Guards are usually the first line of defence for a secure area. Sentinel lymph node biopsy involves identifying the lymph node (or gland) which the breast drains to first. It is the guard to the armpit—the sentinel gland! If cancer cells have breached the axilla and taken up residence, they should at the very least be found in this sentinel node.

Finding the sentinel node (or nodes—there can be several) is done via injection of a radioactive material into the breast and a scan which shows where the node is. At operation the surgeon has a probe to look for this node. Blue dye injected at operation is often used to help this process. If the sentinel node is non-cancerous, it is presumed that the rest of the axilla is too and no further action needs to be taken. If any node contains cancerous cells, axillary clearance is completed—either at the time of initial surgery, or at a second operation once full testing of the sentinel node/s has been undertaken.

Complications such as lymphoedema are very low, but the procedure can be complex and does require specialist expertise. It may not be suitable for all women—especially those with larger tumours, or with tumours in more than one area of the breast.

The operation—what to expect

Before surgery

- Assessment by an anaesthetist prior to surgery to check fitness
- Fast 6 hours prior to surgery (no food or drink)
- Operation site marked by surgeon prior to surgery

> It is very important to discuss what you can expect in the lead up to, on the day of, and after surgery, as well as any concerns, with your surgeon.

After surgery

- Pain relief—usually with simple painkillers such as paracetamol—is needed for a few days
- A drain tube for up to a week, if an axillary clearance or mastectomy has been performed
- If fluid (seroma) builds up under the wound after this it can be drained with a needle
- Physiotherapy and arm exercises

Breast reconstruction

There are various ways of building a new breast and it can be done either at the time of mastectomy or at any stage down the track. Breast reconstruction can also be double-sided should bilateral mastectomy be performed.

> Breast reconstruction can be a crucial step on the path to recovery. Whilst many women choose not to undergo reconstruction, when appropriate, the option should be offered.

Immediate versus delayed reconstruction

Breast reconstruction may involve one or more operations to achieve the final result depending on the method used. Immediate breast reconstruction is when it is done with the mastectomy.

There are a number of benefits to immediate breast reconstruction. It can improve coping and psychological functioning. It can also be technically easier as the breast surgeon can save more skin, and sometimes the nipple and areola, so leading to a better result.

Delayed breast reconstruction can be better for some women. It means the initial surgery is not so extensive, with extra procedures and risks. If radiotherapy is required after mastectomy, it may affect the reconstruction, so women may be advised to wait until after all treatment is completed.

Tissue flap versus implant

There are two basic methods used in breast reconstruction. Implants are the simplest form of reconstruction and can look very good with some body shapes. The other type of reconstruction uses a tissue flap. This is a piece of skin, fat and often muscle brought from elsewhere in the body to build the new breast. The common types of tissue flap used in breast reconstruction are the LD or latissimus dorsi flap taken from the back and the trans-rectus abdominis muscle (TRAM) flap from the tummy.

> It is important to discuss these with the surgeon and treatment team to see which is most suitable for you.

Implant reconstructions are generally done in two stages. Initially, a temporary implant called a tissue expander is placed under the skin and muscle of the chest. Saline is gradually injected to fill it over the weeks following the operation until it has stretched up the muscle and skin around it creating a 'pocket'. At a second operation, a definitive implant, which has a more cosmetically pleasing look and feel, is swapped into this pocket. At this time, a nipple and areola reconstruction can also be performed.

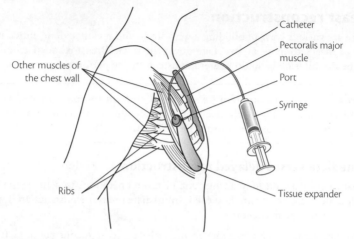

Figure 8.6 A side view of the breast area with an unfilled tissue expander in place.

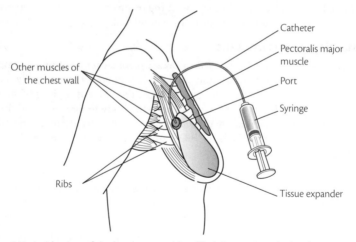

Figure 8.7 A side view of the breast area with a filled tissue expander in place.

Implant reconstructions are the easiest and quickest method but unfortunately do not look ideal on all women.

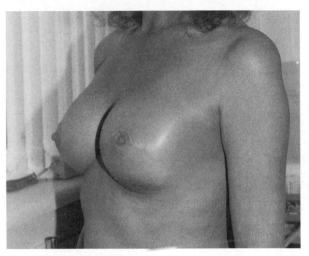

Figure 8.8 An implant reconstruction.

Tissue flap reconstructions are bigger operations but a more realistic shape and feel can be achieved for many women. An LD flap from the back is usually used together with an implant to achieve the correct size match.

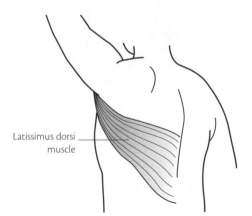

Latissimus dorsi muscle

Figure 8.9 Latissimus dorsi reconstruction: a woman with the latissimus dorsi muscle in place.

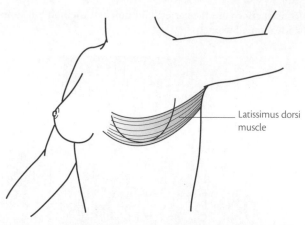

Figure 8.10 Latissimus dorsi reconstruction: a woman with the latissimus dorsi muscle swung forward to recreate the new breast.

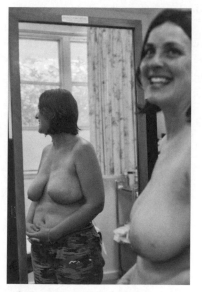

Figure 8.11 A latissimus dorsi reconstruction: front view.

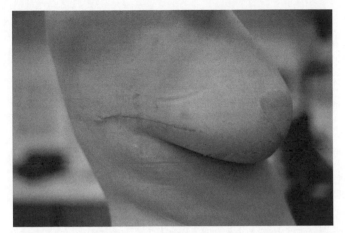

Figure 8.12 A latissimus dorsi reconstruction: back view with the flap scar.

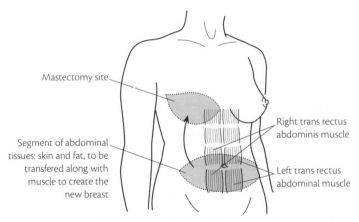

Figure 8.13 Trans-rectus abdominis muscle (TRAM) reconstruction: preparation. (A) The mastectomy site; (B) the right-hand side trans-rectus abdominis muscle; (C) the left-hand side trans-rectus abdominis muscle; (D) a segment of abdominal tissues: skin and fat, to be transferred along with muscle to create the new breast.

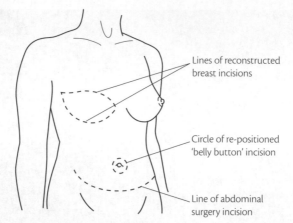

Lines of reconstructed
breast incisions

Circle of re-positioned
'belly button' incision

Line of abdominal
surgery incision

Figure 8.14 A trans-rectus abdominis muscle (TRAM) reconstruction: lines of incision. (A) The lines of reconstructed breast incisions; (B) the circle of the repositioned 'belly button' incision; (C) the line of the abdominal surgery incision.

TRAM flaps from the abdomen provide enough tissue to make a good-sized breast without need for an implant, and can give an excellent cosmetic result. They are not suitable for women who have had previous abdominal surgery or for those who may not do well with a long anaesthetic.

Equalization surgery

When operating on one breast for cancer reasons, it is sometimes useful to perform surgery on the other side too in order to create a matched look. This is known as equalization surgery. It may involve a breast reduction, a one- or double-sided breast lift or even an augmentation (enlargement).

When to avoid surgery

Surgery is not always recommended for breast cancer. If it is not likely to be curative, then it is a lot to put a woman through when there are other treatment options such as chemotherapy, hormonal therapy and radiotherapy. In these situations, surgery is reserved for symptom control—such as if the cancer is becoming a problem by causing ulceration.

On the whole surgery and anaesthesia is very safe, however for very elderly or medically unfit patients it may not be and other treatment such as hormonal drugs are recommended.

Removal of the ovaries

Occasionally, surgical removal of the ovaries (oophorectomy) may make up part of the hormonal treatment of breast cancer in premenopausal patients. There is also a benefit in reducing the risk of both breast and ovarian cancer in a small group of women who have a genetic risk. Oophorectomy can be done either via abdominal surgery or by 'keyhole' (laparoscopic) surgery which means smaller cuts and a quicker recovery. Oophorectomy will cause menopause in premeno- pausal women and any benefits must be weighed up against this. This is dis- cussed in Chapter 11.

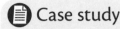 Case study

Beatrice had been diagnosed with a fairly small cancer in her right breast which was detected by a screening mammogram. She had not been able to feel it but the doctor could just feel the lump at about 1cm in size. Beatrice was offered breast-conserving surgery and it was explained she would then need a six-week course of radiotherapy.

Unfortunately Beatrice suffered quite bad arthritis and had undergone a right shoulder replacement two years before. She walked with a stick and at 74, lived alone with no family close by.

She felt coming up to hospital daily for radiotherapy and the pain of having to lift her arm above her head for this, with a stiff shoulder, would make this difficult treatment.

She was not too concerned about the fact of losing her breast—her main con- cern was getting rid of the cancer and returning to as normal a life as possible.

She chose to have a mastectomy and sentinel node biopsy. She did in fact have a small tumour which had not spread to the one lymph node removed and within three weeks she was back to pretty much normal activities. With a prosthesis in her bra she was comfortable with how she looked and happy that no other treatment was needed.

9

Radiotherapy

→ Key Points

♦ Lumpectomy plus breast radiotherapy have similar rates of cure as mastectomy for many patients.

♦ Radiotherapy is virtually *always* recommended after lumpectomy for invasive cancer.

♦ Radiotherapy is sometimes recommended after lumpectomy for DCIS.

♦ Side-effects include local effects on the breast which can last long term and potential effects on other organs.

Radiotherapy is a very useful tool in treating cancer which has been used for over 100 years. Because it uses high-energy radiation, it is a treatment which concerns many people—yet modern radiotherapy utilizes exquisitely accurate technology to target the areas treated and so minimizes side-effects on normal tissues. Breast radiotherapy is, on the whole, very well tolerated and suitable for most women. The few instances where it is not suitable is if the woman has had previous radiotherapy to the area, if she has some skin conditions such as scleroderma, or if she is unable to lie flat for 20 minutes or so with her arm above her head. Because it can only be delivered in specialist centres by very sophisticated equipment, and takes many weeks to deliver, some women who live in remote areas will find this treatment is not right for them.

Breast-conserving therapy

The last 30 years have seen significant improvements in survival for women with breast cancer as well as improvements in the treatments offered. One of the most significant of these has been the widespread introduction of breast-conserving therapy—this means over half of women do not need or do not choose to have a mastectomy, instead having a lumpectomy and radiotherapy, otherwise known as breast-conserving therapy. However, it is important to realize that even though most of the tissue of the breast is conserved the treatment is still to the whole breast—radiotherapy is given to 'mop up' any microscopic cancer cells in the remaining breast tissue.

> **We know from large clinical trials that for most women radiotherapy to the entire breast is important to decrease the chance of the cancer returning in that breast—overall the chance of breast cancer returning in the breast is halved with radiotherapy, and will only occur in a few women.**

Radiotherapy is thus virtually always recommended after a lumpectomy, to the remaining breast tissue on that side and occasionally to the axilla.

What is radiotherapy?

Radiotherapy—or radiation therapy—uses high-powered radiation beams which deliver radioactive particles or X-rays to the targeted tissue in such high doses that they cause death of cells—both normal and cancer cells are killed, but with carefully controlled doses the normal cells are able to recover from this assault whilst the cancer cells cannot. Thus radiation can have side-effects such as scarring of tissue as the normal cells and tissues recover, but the aim is to destroy any remaining microscopic cancer cells in the process.

The first stage of radiotherapy, after meeting the team who will deliver it, and discussing the treatment and side-effects, is the planning session. This uses a simulator machine to mimic where the radiation will be delivered. X-rays and CT scans are done to target very accurately the area the radiation oncologist wishes to treat. The specialist staff will take photographs of the breast.

The area to be treated will be marked with ink and a small tattoo (usually just to the centre of the breast) placed so the radiotherapy can be given each time to the correct area.

Most women having breast or chest wall radiotherapy will require five sessions a week over five to seven weeks—the last two weeks may consist of a 'boost' dose to where the tumour was removed (i.e. the scar). Each treatment takes only a few minutes a day but the woman may need to be in the hospital over half an hour for set-up time and waiting. Once or twice a week a nurse or doctor will check the woman's skin and progress, and occasionally treatment needs to be delayed for a few sessions because of skin reactions.

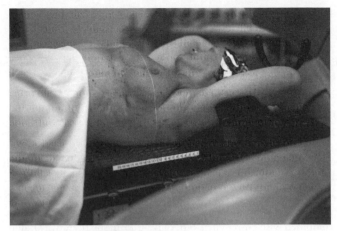

Figure 9.1 A woman having radiotherapy.

Radiotherapy for ductal carcinoma *in situ*

Ductal carcinoma *in situ* (DCIS) is best treated by complete surgical removal, which may be either a mastectomy or lumpectomy. If a lumpectomy is performed radiotherapy may be recommended particularly if the DCIS is over 2cm in size or is high grade (see Chapter 6). There is no evidence that can say definitively which woman with DCIS will benefit or will not benefit from radiotherapy after lumpectomy, so it is best a woman discusses the pros and cons with a radiation oncologist.

> After mastectomy for DCIS, radiotherapy should not be needed.

Radiotherapy for invasive breast cancer

After lumpectomy for invasive cancer radiotherapy to the remaining breast on that side is almost always recommended. This will start anytime from three weeks to around three months after surgery. However, if a woman is going on to have chemotherapy after surgery, radiotherapy is usually delayed until this finishes. Thus the radiotherapy may not start until six or seven months after surgery. This is because combining the two may exacerbate the side-effects of the treatments. Many oncologists will also recommend that hormone drugs such as Tamoxifen or the aromatase inhibitors (Chapter 11) are not given at the same time as chemotherapy, but are started with radiotherapy, although this is still quite controversial.

If there is concern by the medical team that there may be microscopic tumour in the areas around where lymph nodes are situated it is usually suggested that these also undergo irradiation. The penalty for this is a potential for increased side-effects such as lymphoedema (as discussed in Chapter 16).

> **Radiotherapy will halve the chance of cancer returning in the breast or chest wall.**

Advanced and recurrent cancer

Radiotherapy to the breast can only usually be given once as the tissues are not able to tolerate more and may develop ulceration—thus if breast cancer comes back in that breast after lumpectomy, a mastectomy is recommended. Occasionally some extra irradiation can be given if the tumour comes back on the chest wall.

For the small number of women who are first diagnosed with locally advanced cancer and surgery is not possible in the first instance (Chapter 13) radiotherapy can be combined with either chemotherapy or hormone therapy (or all three) to try to shrink the tumour.

Radiotherapy is also used if breast cancer returns in other parts of the body. The most common area for it to be used is in painful bone metastases. This is usually a short course of radiotherapy over five days to two weeks and the aim is not to completely eradicate the cancer (although it may do this) but to alleviate symptoms such as pain and bone collapse. Other areas in which breast cancer can recur and to which radiotherapy treatment can be very helpful include the brain and the lungs.

Side-effects of radiotherapy
Skin and breast tissue

During radiotherapy the breast usually feels tight and may be tender. This is usually accompanied by a pinkness of the skin like sunburn, but the skin may be very red with some temporary skin peeling with blistering and weeping. This usually clears up within a few weeks of radiotherapy but there is often some residual skin change lasting many years or forever. This is usually mild— the breast feels a bit firmer and is sensitive to touch. The skin in the treated area may also be a little darker than normal—like a permanent suntan. This occurs more in people with olive skin. However, it can be more severe with a 'woodiness' to the breast tissues and some puckering of the skin. Unfortunately women with larger breasts are most likely to have worse effects in the longer term. Smoking, sun exposure and some health problems such as diabetes can also make the skin problems worse.

The radiation therapists and nurses, as well as the radiation oncologists, can give good advice about how to minimize these effects. We suggest you use mild, non-perfumed soap and a recommended moisturiser, avoid the sun and use suncream when you are in it, and avoid deodorant during treatment.

Side-effects of radiotherapy include:

- Skin change like a sunburn
- Pigmentation of skin
- Woodiness of the breast tissue
- Fatigue
- Depression
- Rarely damage to lungs or extremely rarely second cancers

Surrounding tissues

There may be some temporary stiffness in the muscles around the chest. Radiotherapy to the lymph nodes can also contribute to lymphoedema (see Chapter 16). Good physiotherapy can help with these.

The whole body

Many women will feel tired during radiotherapy and this can last. Regular exercise will help with this. Depression is also common—this is treatable and should be discussed with the care team who can offer help and advice.

Very rarely radiotherapy can damage other body organs such as the lungs, causing fibrosis or extremely rarely on the left side, the heart. Another extremely rare long-term problem is a second cancer called a sarcoma.

It is important to discuss side-effects with the treatment team.

New types of radiotherapy
Partial breast irradiation

Of the few breast cancers that return in the breast after lumpectomy, most do so close to where the original tumour was situated. Thus there is a logical argument that it is this region of the breast that requires radiotherapy, and some women may not need the rest of the breast irradiated. We still do not know if this is the case, and so a number of studies around the world are trying to answer this question. There are a variety of techniques being tried which target radiotherapy to just one area of the breast. The advantage of most of them is that they cut down the number of days needed for radiotherapy to anything from a one-off dose (for intra-operative radiotherapy) to a few days (for devices such as the Mammosite device and brachytherapy). However, they are still experimental and we do not know if they will prove as good as (or perhaps better than) conventional radiotherapy until the studies are complete. Nor do we yet know which patients they may be best for.

Intensity-modulated radiotherapy

This type of treatment allows better focus of the radiotherapy to where it is most needed. It is not known yet if this will lead to better control of a breast cancer, and thus a lower chance of recurrence, nor if it will help alleviate side effects, but it is a promising technique that a number of centres around the world are studying.

📄 Case study

Margaret is a 65-year-old woman who presented with a lump in her right breast, directly under her nipple and pulling the nipple in.

This was shown on mammogram, ultrasound and needle biopsy to be a cancer measuring 5cm in size. The surgeon who first examined her in the breast clinic also thought he could feel some enlarged lymph glands under the arm and a needle biopsy of these also showed cancer cells in them. The surgeon arranged other tests including CT scans and a bone scan and these did not show any spread of breast cancer to other organs.

Margaret underwent a mastectomy and axillary clearance and the week after surgery she discussed the pathology results with the surgeon. This showed a 4cm Grade 2 lobular cancer of the breast with 5 of the 15 lymph nodes removed involved with cancer. The tumour was oestrogen and progesterone receptor positive and cerbB2 receptor negative. Margaret was a fit and well retired and widowed teacher who was a keen bowls enthusiast.

She underwent six months of chemotherapy, and actually managed to come through this very well—she did lose her hair but had been able to re-start her bowls about a month after surgery – this seemed to help with the fatigue of chemotherapy and the support of her bowls club and team members helped her through the treatment.

3 weeks after finishing chemotherapy she started a 7 week course of radiotherapy to the chest wall, under the arm and above the collarbone on the right. She had few skin problems but found, on top of the residual tiredness of chemotherapy, coming up to the hospital every day was exhausting. However, timing this so she could get a lift with a friend in the middle of the day when traffic was lightest helped, as did planning a rest after treatment.

After radiotherapy Margaret started on Tamoxifen tablets and came for regular check-ups with both the surgeon and oncologists.

Unfortunately she did develop some mild lymphoedema about a year after surgery – she felt this may have been related to some insect bites on the arm. This was improved with the help of the physiotherapist, but did stop her bowls for a season.

10

Chemotherapy

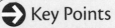 **Key Points**

- Chemotherapy is treatment that kills dividing cells, and aims to target the rapidly dividing cancer cells.

- Most chemotherapy regimens last for four to six months, and usually involve injections every three or four weeks with a stay in hospital for a day of that time, plus tablets in between.

- Blood tests will help monitor whether the body's normal cells (such as blood cells) have recovered enough between each round of treatment to have a full dose of the next treatment.

- Side-effects are due to the effects of chemotherapy on other normal body cells, in particular the bone marrow and hair.

What is chemotherapy?

Chemotherapy is drug treatment given usually via a vein into the bloodstream and as tablets. A few chemotherapy drugs are tablets only. All these drugs target dividing cells causing them to stop dividing and self-destruct. Another name is cytotoxic therapy, which literally means killing cells. Although both normal cells and cancer cells are affected, most normal body cells are much better able to recover (or are more resistant) so most of the cells that die will be cancer cells. Treatments are given over a number of courses as each course will kill more and more of the cancer cells. This also gives the body's normal cells a chance to recover between cycles.

The normal cells that are most affected are those with a rapid turnover—such as hair follicle cells (hence hair loss) and the bone marrow where blood cells are made (hence some of the other complications such as anaemia and low white cell and platelet counts).

Assessing who should have chemotherapy

Chemotherapy overall reduces the chance of breast cancer returning by about a third. However, when and for whom it is used will vary between patients. It is essentially a decision based upon the risks and presumed benefits of chemotherapy. The decision by the cancer team to recommend chemotherapy depends on a number of factors:

- How aggressive the patient's tumour appears clinically and under the microscope (the tumour stage)
- How much the tumour is likely to respond to treatments other than chemotherapy (i.e. hormonal therapy—see Chapter 11)
- A patient's age and whether the woman herself is fit enough to undergo chemotherapy
- The choice of the woman herself based on the risks and benefits.

The benefits of chemotherapy have been worked out from information gained from doing clinical trials—these are often very large studies (up to thousands of patients) where the patients have agreed to enter a study where two treatments are compared for both how effective they are and the side-effects they may cause. A useful tool in helping make a decision is an online website called adjuvantonline.com which is developed and updated by oncologists, and can give some general information on the benefits of chemotherapy as well as hormone therapy. Because new information is being gained all the time from such studies, it is important that patients discuss all potential treatments with the medical oncologist.

Options for treatment

Most chemotherapy treatment will consist of more than one drug—either given together or sequentially. This is because different drugs target different actions of the cell so kill in different ways.

The actual combination given to an individual woman will depend on many factors including the type of breast cancer, the age and fitness of the patient, the side-effect profile of the drugs and what side-effects the woman can tolerate and wishes to tolerate for the slight differences in effectiveness of the drugs, the experience and preferences of the treating oncologist—and even cost and the availability within the hospital prescribing system.

So, for example, a chemotherapy treatment including anthracylcine drugs is somewhat more effective than the more traditional combinations but may have more side-effects. A patient needs to discuss this in detail with her medical oncologist to fully understand the decisions made and her potential side-effects and benefits.

Timing of chemotherapy

Chemotherapy is most often given after surgery to the breast and axilla but before radiotherapy or hormone therapy, if these are required. This is called adjuvant chemotherapy. It may also be given as a first line treatment, before surgery or radiotherapy, and is then called neo-adjuvant chemotherapy. This is most commonly when the tumour is large in relation to the breast (locally advanced breast cancer) and the aim of the chemotherapy is to shrink the tumour thus possibly allowing breast-conserving surgery. In some women the tumour is not amenable to surgery when they are first diagnosed (because the tumour is stuck to the chest wall or of an inflammatory type) so the chemotherapy is aimed at making surgery by mastectomy possible.

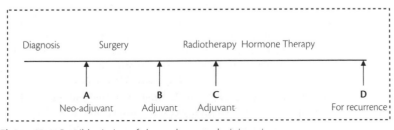

Figure 10.1 Possible timing of chemotherapy administration.

Chemotherapy is also given to many women with recurrent cancer, particularly if it has spread to other organs in the body. This is discussed in Chapter 13.

Having chemotherapy

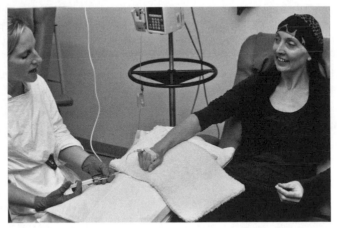

Figure 10.2 A patient having chemotherapy.

Chemotherapy needs to be prescribed and supervised by a specialist oncologist, although for patients in rural areas where it is hard to access specialists regularly, some drugs can be given by non-specialists or nurses, if this is agreed by the medical oncologist.

Treatment is usually in a specialist chemotherapy clinic in the hospital, where the patient is admitted for the day. Blood tests prior to treatment ensure that the bone marrow is producing enough blood cells to make treatment safe, and then the drugs are given usually into a vein (this is called intravenously or IV) over half an hour to a few hours, depending on the type of drugs. Some treatment combinations also involve tablets.

Chemotherapy nurses will administer the drugs and also be an invaluable source of information and help with side-effects. Chemotherapy is given in 'cycles': a day of the chemotherapy treatment followed by two to four weeks of no treatment to allow the body time to recover, then another dose of chemotherapy. This will last for four to six cycles usually equating to three to six months.

> **Chemotherapy is prescribed and coordinated by a medical oncologist, although it can be given by a specially trained nurse or GP.**

Side-effects and complications

Unfortunately virtually all patients having chemotherapy will experience some side-effects, although for many this will be tolerable—many women can continue to work, do regular exercise and hobbies and even continue pregnancy through chemotherapy.

Common side-effects include fatigue, nausea, a sore mouth and hair loss, although specific drugs will have their own specific complications. It is difficult to predict who will get side-effects and to what extent—however most women find the side-effects do get somewhat worse over the course of the treatments.

Any side-effects, even mild ones, should be reported to the nursing and medical teams as most can be managed very well.

> ### Common side-effects of chemotherapy
>
> - Nausea and vomiting
> - Fatigue
> - Hair loss
> - Diarrhoea or constipation
> - Weight gain or loss
> - Mouth ulcers
> - Dry and cracked skin
> - Feeling a bit vague ('chemo fog')
> - Depression
> - Unpleasant taste in the mouth, especially with some foods

Less common side-effects of chemotherapy

- Red palms and feet
- Tingling hands and feet
- Infections—this may be due to low white blood cell counts and may require a stay in hospital
- Bruising easily

Rarer side-effects of chemotherapy

- Urinary infections
- Heart problems
- Allergic reactions

Chemotherapy often causes early menopause and subsequent loss of fertility in pre-menopausal women and is discussed in detail in Chapter 16.

New treatments

The last decade has seen an exponential increase in new drug treatments available for breast cancer. Some of these are new chemotherapy agents and many of these, such as the taxanes, have proven very effective treatments and are now part of the standard management for many women with breast cancer.

A real goal of finding new chemotherapy agents is to discover those which are more efficacious but also those better tolerated, and perhaps in tablet form, such as capecitabine. Because chemotherapy works best as a combination of agents there is also much research going on into the best combination of the dozen or more drugs currently in common use. Many patients will be invited to join clinical trials of new agents and new combinations (Chapter 12).

11

Hormones and breast cancer

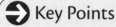 Key Points

- Two-thirds of breast cancers grow in response to the female hormone oestrogen.

- HRT and the Pill slightly increase a woman's chance of developing breast cancer, and are not recommended after breast cancer diagnosis.

- Hormonal therapies for breast cancer such as Tamoxifen and the aromatase inhibitors are very effective at decreasing the chance of the cancer returning.

- These hormonal therapies may have side-effects, in particular menopause symptoms.

Previous chapters have discussed surgical, radiation and chemotherapy treatment for breast cancer. For a large majority of women with breast cancer, hormone treatment will play an important role in their management. This chapter discusses not only hormone treatments for breast cancer but also how hormones either made in a woman's body or which she may take, such as the Pill or HRT, may influence the development of a breast cancer.

The majority of breast cancers grow under the influence of hormones—most notably oestrogen. This has significantly changed the way we view HRT and even the oral contraceptive pill, which both contain oestrogen and/or progesterone. Treatment options utilizing the hormone-responsive nature of breast cancer have advanced our ability to successfully combat and cure these cancers in appropriate patients. Like chemotherapy, hormonal therapy is a form of systemic, or full body, treatment. Whereas surgery and radiotherapy target specific sites of disease in the body, systemic therapies, travelling via the bloodstream, can lead to destruction of cancer cells anywhere in the body.

Oestrogen

Oestrogen is a hormone made predominantly in the ovaries, from puberty and the onset of menstruation (menarche) until menopause. Smaller amounts of oestrogen are also made in the body's fat from adrenal gland hormones under influence from the enzyme, aromatase. At menopause, whilst the levels of oestrogen drop markedly, there will always be some ongoing production.

The connection, if not the exact nature of the relationship, between oestrogen and breast cancer has long been known. As discussed in Chapter 2, women with reduced exposure to periods of higher oestrogen production have a lower risk of developing breast cancer. This includes women who start their periods later than usual, those who have their first child before 30, those who breast-feed for extended periods and those in whom menopause comes on early either naturally or after surgical removal of the ovaries. By contrast, women who have used the oral contraceptive pill or HRT, which both contain oestrogen and/or progesterone, are at an increased risk of breast cancer. All of these factors may be associated with the increase in breast cancer seen over the past five decades, particularly in the West, where there has been a trend towards earlier onset of puberty, later child rearing and increased use of the pill and HRT.

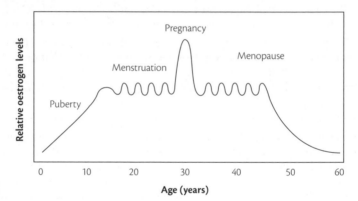

Figure 11.1 Oestrogen production levels according to age.

The role of oestrogen

- Over two-thirds of breast cancers and particularly those in post-menopausal women, grow under the influence of oestrogen.

- The cells making up these cancers have oestrogen and/or progesterone binding sites known as oestrogen and progesterone *receptors*.

- We can test cancers for these receptors on the cancer specimen which helps plan which patients are likely to respond to anti-oestrogen medications.

Hormone replacement therapy

There has been a lot in the press over the past few years about the risk of taking hormone replacement therapy with regard to developing breast cancer. This has largely been due to two studies—the Women's Health Initiative (WHI) by the World Health Organization (WHO) and the Million Women Study undertaken in the United Kingdom. Both studies showed a small increase in breast cancer rates among women taking combined hormone replacement therapy—that is containing an oestrogen and progesterone. In the WHI study, the risk only became significant once women had taken four or more years of combined hormone replacement therapy. It showed no increase in breast cancer rates amongst women taking oestrogen-only hormone replacement therapy, although this finding is at odds with the conclusions reached in other trials, including the Million Women Study.

Whilst use of combined hormonal replacement therapy beyond four years appears to increase the risk of breast cancer, ceasing hormonal supplementation brings that risk back down to normal levels within about five years.

> Any decision to commence or cease hormone replacement therapy must be a considered one between a patient and her doctor/s, taking into account the patient's existing breast cancer risk and the level of symptoms associated with menopause.

Certainly, in a woman of average breast cancer risk with debilitating menopausal symptoms, it seems reasonable to try a course of hormone replacement therapy for less than five years, at which stage things should be reassessed to weigh up the increasing risks of ongoing usage versus the benefits to the woman's daily lifestyle.

It should be noted here that in addition to increasing breast cancer risk, hormone replacement therapy has also been linked with a small increase in cardiovascular problems such as heart attacks, stroke and blood clots elsewhere. Obviously, this also needs to be weighed up in any treatment decision process.

Oral contraceptive pill

So what of the Pill, which contains varying combinations of oestrogens and progesterone? It is very possible that there is an increased risk of breast cancer with use of pills containing oestrogen. Whilst much research has looked at this, no definite conclusion has been reached. This is because any small increased risk the Pill poses will be minute considering how rarely breast cancer occurs in young women of the age group likely to be on the Pill.

> This tiny increase in the risk of breast cancer should not be of concern for young women on the pill.

Hormone replacement therapy, by contrast, is targeted at postmenopausal women whose ages are largely above 45; breast cancer risk climbs with age meaning that postmenopausal women are the ones most at risk already and are therefore more 'susceptible' to added risks such as with HRT. The risk from the pill and HRT drops back to normal within two years of stopping the pill.

Pregnancy

Given the hormonal changes that occur during pregnancy, it is reasonable to ask what effect this may have on both the risk of developing breast cancer and on a cancer itself should it come on during pregnancy. Regarding the risk of breast cancer a full-term pregnancy under the age of 30 is protective against developing breast cancer, and the total number of pregnancies adds additional benefit.

Pregnancy during and after breast cancer is discussed in Chapter 15.

Breastfeeding

As mentioned in Chapter 2, breastfeeding is also known to reduce a woman's overall risk of developing breast cancer via the hormonal changes that take place. The reduction in risk seems to increase along with the number of years spent breastfeeding. So what does this mean for a woman deciding whether or not she will breastfeed her child and if so, for how long? In reality, the effect on an individual woman's risk of developing breast cancer is likely to be very small. To look at that another way, in 1000 women who breastfed for a year versus 1000 who did not, there may be four additional women who develop breast cancer over their lifetime in the group who did not breastfeed. It is not therefore something which should really come into the decision-making process when there are a myriad of other, more significant issues to take into account.

Hormonal therapy for breast cancer

Manipulating the hormonal aspect of breast cancer has proven to be a powerful way in which to treat it. There are now various drugs available for use in selected patients, giving us many hormonal treatment options. First and foremost, however, a breast cancer must be deemed 'hormone-responsive'. This is done by testing cancer cells for both oestrogen and progesterone receptors, and can be done on a needle biopsy tissue specimen or the surgically excised cancer. Whilst most premenopausal cancers are hormone receptor negative, or hormone insensitive, overall almost 75% of breast cancers do exhibit some hormone sensitivity, making hormonal treatment a useful option.

Question to ask the doctor: Which hormone therapy is best for me?

This will depend on whether a woman has gone through menopause or not, and what side-effects the drugs may cause her, as well as which drug is most effective for her cancer.

How hormonal therapies work

Hormonal treatments mostly work by either reducing the overall amount of oestrogen in the body or by stopping the oestrogen present exerting its usual effect. The result for hormone-responsive breast cancer cells is that they are starved of the oestrogen they require to help them grow. Other, non-cancerous body tissues may miss out on the good effect of oestrogen due to the cancer treatment, leading to not so desirable effects. In fact, whilst hormonal treatments are usually easier for patients to take than chemotherapy, there are still some significant side-effects, which need to be considered. This is particularly important given that hormonal treatment is usually given over at least five years and as such can have a very significant effect on a woman's life.

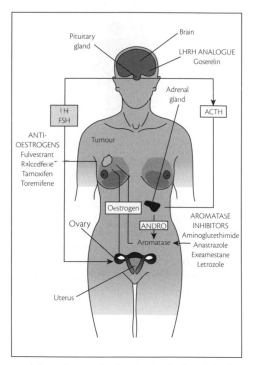

Figure 11.2 Hormonal therapies: mode of action in the female body.

LH, luteinizing hormone; FSH, follicle-stimulating hormone; ACTH, adrenocorticotrophic hormone; ANDRO, androstenedione.

Side-effects of hormonal therapies

Most commonly, women may experience symptoms similar to those of menopause. Hot flushes and sweats, mood and sleep disturbance, reduced interest in sex and vaginal dryness are common complaints. Women still getting periods may notice a change in their cycle or even a complete stop of menstruation. Symptoms are usually worst when treatment is started and often settle down within weeks to months. For those women who are still suffering significant problems after this initial period, it is imperative to address the issues rather than simply stopping the treatment—this can lead to an increased risk of relapse. As hormonal treatments are more commonly used, the side-effects are better understood, giving more ability to effectively manage them. This is discussed in Chapter 16.

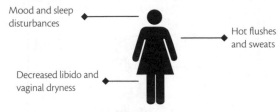

Mood and sleep disturbances

Hot flushes and sweats

Decreased libido and vaginal dryness

Figure 11.3 Hormonal therapy side-effects.

Tamoxifen

How it works

Premenopausal women with hormone receptor positive cancers will generally be offered Tamoxifen. Tamoxifen is a tablet taken once daily, usually for 5 years. It is absorbed into the bloodstream and travels to any breast cancer cells where it binds onto the oestrogen receptors mentioned earlier. With Tamoxifen effectively blocking these spots, the cancer cells are starved of the oestrogen they need to grow. Many other cell types around the body also have oestrogen receptors, meaning that the effect of Tamoxifen may be beyond just the cancer cells.

Side-effects

Depending on the cell type, Tamoxifen may simply block the oestrogen effect (as in breast cancer cells) or in some tissues, by binding at the receptor, it may exert an oestrogen-like stimulatory effect. Tamoxifen acting in this way can stimulate growth of the uterine (womb) lining. Occasionally, women may experience abnormal vaginal bleeding as a result. In rare situations, there is even the possibility of uterine cancer. It has been estimated that for women on Tamoxifen, the additional risk of developing uterine cancer beyond that for other women equates to about 1 in 1000 per year. There is also a small increased risk of blood clots such as deep venous thrombosis (DVT) in the legs and pelvis and clots causing stroke. Compared to the potentially large benefit of treating their breast cancer, most women find these unlikely side-effects an acceptable risk.

Ovarian suppression and ablation

In some premenopausal women, there may be a benefit in turning the ovaries off—either temporarily via medication or permanently with radiotherapy or surgical removal. The idea behind this is to reduce any oestrogen in the body as much as possible, as the oestrogen may promote breast cancer growth. It is only relevant in premenopausal women, as post menopause, the ovaries no longer produce oestrogen.

How it works

Ovarian suppression means switching off the ovaries with medication. The commonly used class of drugs for this purpose are the gonadotrophin-releasing hormone analogues (GnRH analogues). GnRH analogues trick the pituitary gland into reducing production of luteinizing hormone (LH), which is required by the ovaries to drive oestrogen production. A drug-induced lack of LH puts the ovaries to 'sleep'; a kind of early but temporary menopause whilst the drug is used. Goserelin (or Zoladex) is the most common GnRH analogue in breast cancer and is usually administered monthly by an injection under the skin. It is mostly recommended for premenopausal women with more advanced cancers where relapse is a greater possibility. Sometimes, Goserelin is given with chemotherapy in an attempt to protect the ovaries, and hence a woman's fertility, from the chemotherapy effects. The idea is that by suppressing the ovaries whilst chemotherapy is in the system, they may be less likely to be permanently shut down by the chemotherapy. How well this works is not clear at this stage.

Ovarian ablation refers to the permanent shutting down of the ovaries. This can be achieved by surgical removal of the ovaries or by radiotherapy to the ovaries. Some women prefer this to, potentially, years of monthly injections.

Side-effects

Induced menopause will be associated with temporary or permanent loss of fertility, predisposition to osteoporosis and other long-term effects. These issues will be addressed later in this book in Chapter 16. Sometimes, the sudden reduction in oestrogen levels after ovarian ablation can bring on quite severe menopausal symptoms. Usually, these will settle down in time.

In a premenopausal woman who it is felt will benefit from maximal possible oestrogen suppression and who is past her childbearing years, ovarian ablation should be considered. There may also be some additional benefit in surgical removal of the ovaries in some women who have a family history of breast or ovarian cancer as they may be at an increased risk of developing ovarian cancer themselves.

Table 11.1 Comparison of removing ovaries versus using drugs to suppress ovarian function

Ovarian ablation	Ovarian suppression
Permanent menopause	Usually temporary menopause
Permanent loss of fertility	Fertility may return
One treatment only	Monthly injections for 2–5 years
Removes the risk of developing ovarian cancer	May decrease the risk of developing ovarian cancer

Aromatase inhibitors

Postmenopausal patients with hormone-sensitive cancers can be considered differently due to the fact that the ovaries are not active. Compared with pre-menopausal patients, there is less oestrogen. This opens up other, potentially more effective, treatment options. Removal of the ovaries or otherwise shutting them down obviously becomes unnecessary. The most common type of drugs used in this group of patients is the aromatase inhibitors: Anastrazole, Exemestane and Letrozole. Like Tamoxifen, they are given once daily, usually for five years.

How they work

These drugs inactivate the hormone, aromatase, thus stopping the conversion of adrenal gland hormones into oestrogen. So whilst Tamoxifen stops oestrogen working at the breast cancer cell, the aromatase inhibitor drugs aim to reduce the total amount of oestrogen circulating in the body.

Side-effects

There is mounting evidence that aromatase inhibitors are more effective than Tamoxifen in reducing relapse from breast cancer and are also at least as effective as Tamoxifen in bringing about long-term cure. There are, however some specific side-effects associated with aromatase inhibitors that may still mean Tamoxifen is a better choice for some postmenopausal women. In particular, aromatase inhibitors can cause quite marked bone and joint pain. In some women, these pains can be quite difficult to treat although there are various strategies used to deal with the problem including simple pain medications or anti-inflammatory gels, swapping between different aromatase inhibitors or even taking a break from the medication for a period of time. Osteoporosis and bone fractures are also increased in women on these drugs over long periods of time. We will discuss this further in Chapter 16.

Table 11.2 Comparison of the benefits and drawbacks of Tamoxifen versus aromatase inhibitors

	Tamoxifen	Aromatase inhibitors
Benefits	Effective anti-cancer drug Mechanism of action and side-effects well understood	Slightly more effective anti-cancer drug
Drawbacks	May develop blood clots such as deep venous thrombosis Possible irregular vaginal bleeding Small risk womb cancer	May develop joint pains May lead to bone thinning and an increased risk of osteoporosis and bone fractures with long-term use Can only be used after menopause

Prevention of breast cancer

As mentioned in Chapter 2, methods used to hormonally manipulate breast cancers can also have a protective effect in avoiding future breast cancers.

> **Women who undergo ovarian ablation as part of their treatment halve their risk of developing a future new breast cancer.**

Whilst this is not necessarily a reason to undergo ovarian ablation, given that the risk of future breast cancer may be small compared to the consequences of early menopause, it is a nice additional benefit of the treatment. Similarly, treatment with Tamoxifen or an aromatase inhibitor will lower the risk of future breast cancers. Considerable effort has been put into determining whether or not it is reasonable to treat some healthy women with these drugs prophylactically in an attempt to lower their risk of developing breast cancer in the first place. It is a difficult question given that the benefit would need to be quite significant to justify using medications which have side-effects in healthy women who may be unlikely to ever develop breast cancer. Certainly, there may be a place for this in specific groups of women at particularly high risk of breast cancer. There is no consensus on this currently.

📄 Case study

Brenda is a 57-year-old book keeper who had breast cancer diagnosed through the breast screening programme. She had never felt a lump or any symptoms, and had never had any previous breast problems.

She had a hysterectomy eight years prior to her breast cancer for heavy periods, and after her surgery had developed a deep vein thrombosis.

Brenda is a slim woman whose mother had had fairly severe osteoporosis which had made her bed-bound at the end of her life. Brenda was aware she was at risk of this so kept in good health, exercised regularly and took calcium supplements. She had given up smoking ten years before on the advice of her GP that this could contribute to the development of osteoporosis.

Brenda had a hook wire localized excision of the cancer and sentinel node biopsy (see Chapter 8). The surgeon informed her the pathology showed an 18 mm grade 2 invasive ductal cancer with no involvement of the lymph ode and the tumour was hormone-receptor positive.

She made an excellent recovery from surgery and went on to have breast radiotherapy. She was advised a hormonal therapy would decrease her risks of recurrence by 5 to 10% over the next 10 years and she wished to consider this. Tamoxifen first seemed a good option – she was keen to take a drug which had been tried and tested over many years and as she had had a hysterectomy she did not need to worry about the possibility of bleeding from the womb. However she mentioned her DVT history and her surgeon suggested she consider an aromatase inhibitor instead.

Brenda was worried as these may make osteoporosis worse – however she had a bone density scan and this showed her bones to be good for her age, so she went ahead with the aromatase inhibitor and arranged yearly bone density monitoring.

This fell a little but with a good diet, exercise and calcium and vitamin D supplements she was able to keep her bones healthy – and did not get any other side effects.

12

New drug treatments

> ### ➡ Key Points
>
> ◆ Targeted drugs are those that attack the single part of a cancer cell and so selectively destroy these cells.
>
> ◆ Herceptin targets the 15% or so of breast cancers that have the growth receptor Her2.
>
> ◆ Other targeted drugs affect other growth receptors and the tumour blood supply.
>
> ◆ Newer chemotherapy and hormonal drugs are being developed which will be more specific and hopefully more effective with less side-effects.

This chapter discusses some of the newer treatments for breast cancer and tries to look into the near future to predict what may be available for breast cancer patients over the next few years.

Targeted drugs

The changes in cells which cause them to become cancerous include a whole series of faults in the genetic machinery which lead to the checks and balances being upset—thus the cells multiply unchecked, grow in abnormal patterns and eventually the cancer cells spread to other parts of the body. It seems ideal therefore to develop treatments that do not just 'blindly' damage all of the body's cells but which target and destroy the cells with these gene faults, that is the cancer cells.

An enormous amount of scientific research has gone on, and continues to go on, into exactly how cells become cancerous, and this has now begun to lead to real advances in treatments. These treatments are called targeted drugs.

Targeted drugs have been developed which seek out and tear down a variety of processes in the cancer cells, including molecules on their surface which allow them to grow unchecked (growth factor receptors) and their ability to develop their own blood supply (anti-angiogenic agents).

In many ways hormonal treatments such as Tamoxifen are targeted drugs—they target cancers which are hormone-receptor positive. These drugs are discussed in Chapter 11.

Trastuzumab (Herceptin®)

Around 15–20% of breast cancers make an excess of molecules on the cell surface which allows them to grow, invade and develop a blood supply of their own. This molecule is known as the Her2 growth factor receptor, and cells with excess of this are said to over-express this receptor and be 'Her2 positive' or 'cerbB2 positive'.

The drug trastuzumab, or Herceptin as it is commonly known, attaches specifically to these receptors and stops them working. The drug is only effective in the tumours which over-express the receptor, and this can be tested on a tumour specimen by the pathologist.

Clinical trials have shown that for the 20% or so of women with tumours which over-express the receptor, Herceptin will improve the chance of tumour not returning by around a third. This is particularly important as these tumours often seem to be aggressive and resistant to some other treatments.

Herceptin is used both in early breast cancer and in women with metastatic disease. In the setting of early breast cancer it is usually combined with chemotherapy and often given for one year—by weekly or three-weekly intravenous injection, which takes around 90 minutes. Many women will experience mild flu-like symptoms whilst on the drug but overall it is very well tolerated. A small percentage of women can develop heart problems on Herceptin and it is therefore important to get a heart scan prior to starting the drug.

Herceptin is an antibody, so, like the body's own antibodies which are part of the immune system, it causes the immune system to kill the affected cells. This is a kind of immune, or biological therapy.

Bevacizumab (Avastin®)

This is a drug which blocks the growth of new blood vessels or angiogenesis. Cancer cells make a growth factor which stimulates angiogenesis, called vascular endothelial growth factor (VEGF), and Avastin blocks this, making cells die and be more vulnerable to chemotherapy.

To date it has only been used in advanced breast cancer in combination with chemotherapy, although it is under clinical trial for a number of settings. It is given by intravenous injection over an hour every few weeks. It can cause high blood pressure but other more serious side-effects are possible and need to be discussed with an oncologist.

Avastin is also an immune therapy.

Lapatinib (Tykerb®)

This drug again works against Her2-positive cells, but this time it interferes with the signals inside the cells (called kinases) which are promoting growth and multiplication of the cell. Unlike Herceptin and Avastin it is not an antibody but a chemical.

Tykerb is most often used for women with Her2-positive metastatic cancer whose tumours are not responding to other drugs such as Herceptin. It is a tablet usually given with the chemotherapy tablet Xeloda (capecitabine). It does not often have serious side-effects but can cause diarrhoea and vomiting. Fatigue can be a real problem for many women with advanced breast cancer, and some of this may be due to the medication.

New chemotherapy drugs

There continues to be much research around the best combination of chemotherapy drugs, the best doses of the drugs, how they should be combined with the targeted drugs discussed above, and how best to minimize the side-effects of these drugs. PARP inhibitors constitute one new group of drugs and are described here. There will no doubt be many others in development over the next few years.

PARP inhibitors

A new type of chemotherapy drug called PARP inhibitors have recently been discovered which use a mechanism of action which specifically targets cancer cells that have lost their ability to repair their faulty genes (DNA). These tumours are the type found in women who carry an inherited gene fault in the *BRCA 1* or *BRCA 2* gene (see Chapter 2). PARP inhibitors selectively kill cells where this form of DNA repair is absent and so are highly effective in killing *BRCA* tumour cells and other similar tumour cells. Normal cells are largely unaffected by the drug as they still possess this crucial DNA repair mechanism.

These drugs are still in the early test phases for both breast and ovarian cancer in women who have *BRCA* gene faults.

New hormonal drugs

The aromatase inhibitors have now become standard treatment for many postmenopausal women with hormone receptor positive breast cancer, and are discussed in detail in Chapter 11. Research is currently underway into how long these drugs should be used for, and whether a sequence of different hormone drugs may be best.

Other hormone drugs are also being developed. The drug fulvestrant (Faslodex®) completely blocks oestrogen receptors and is used in some women with metastatic breast cancer. It is a monthly injection.

In pre-menopausal women with hormone receptor positive tumours, stopping the ovaries working with drugs such as goserelin (Zoladex®) or triptorelin has been shown to be of additional benefit in reducing the chance of the disease returning.

Clinical trials

Whereas most advances in medicine have come from the laboratory and from experiments in cell cultures or mice, it is vitally important these advances are tested in humans with the disease. Thus clinical trials are the type of research performed which tells us if one treatment is better than another. Clinical trials are carefully worked out studies which have to be approved by ethics committees and scientific committees at each hospital where they are being run.

Participating in a clinical trial is a generous act which may not be of any specific advantage to the individual. However, many women with breast cancer feel it is important to do so, as they will be helping the next generation of women with the disease. It also means a woman may receive a newer treatment, and we know that the close monitoring and follow-up patients receive in clinical trials, along with the fact that they are usually conducted by centres with a specific interest in the disease, means patients in trials tend to have better outcomes than those not in them.

However, the new treatment being tested in the trial may not be more effective than the standard treatment and may have more side-effects. A clinical trial has the treatments randomized so neither the patient nor her doctor chooses which treatment she will receive, and she may receive the new treatment or the standard one.

> It is important to weigh up the benefits and disadvantages of taking part in a clinical trial—if you choose not to join your treatment and care will remain the best standard available and it will not affect how your doctor treats you. You may also decide to leave a trial at any time and go back on to standard treatment without giving a reason.

Your confidentiality and privacy should be guaranteed if you participate in clinical research—you can check with your doctor and on the information sheet and consent form for the trial that the trail complies with all privacy agreements which are made by law.

Things to consider before going into a clinical trial

± By choosing to join a trial you will be contributing to the effort to combat cancer.

± The treatment you receive in a trial will be at least the best available.

± You cannot choose which treatment you receive in a trial.

± You may receive treatment you would not otherwise have access to.

± You will have close monitoring in a trial, and any additional tests or treatment should not cost you money.

± You have the right not to participate in a trial or to withdraw at any time without giving a reason.

The next decade . . .

There continue to be very exciting developments in new drug treatments—agents which block all parts of the hugely complex cell pathways which make a cancer cell act like it does. There is even the possibility of vaccines for established cancer—and perhaps in 20 or 30 years vaccines to prevent it.

A very real advance which will be important in the next five to ten years is the ability of the pathologists to characterise the molecular fingerprint of a cancer—to actually look at precisely what pathways have gone wrong, so allowing the precise combination of drugs to be given which will target these pathways—maybe even reversing some of the changes rather than just destroying the cells.

Already some of this new diagnostic technology is available in the form of a test called molecular profiling or a gene array. These are tests done on the tumour specimen after surgical removal which may help give clues as to what *genes* are malfunctioning in the tumour and so how best to treat the cancer. The current challenge is figuring out how this new technology fits in with current pathology techniques—so again clinical trials are testing this.

Most new treatments for cancer are trialled first in patients with advanced disease as it is here that we can measure any effects more easily, and it is hoped that any benefits from new treatments may be gained by patients with these cancers. Advanced disease is discussed in the next chapter.

📄 Case study

Beth is a 36-year-old who developed breast cancer four years ago. It was treated at the time with a mastectomy and axillary clearance, along with chemotherapy. Her tumour did not have receptors for either oestrogen or Her2 (she was told it was a triple negative tumour).

Beth had been adopted and although she knew her birth mother she did not know much about her relatives at the time of diagnosis. She subsequently discovered that she had had an aunt with breast cancer in her thirties, so Beth underwent gene testing and was found to have a *BRCA1* gene fault.

Beth was contemplating having a mastectomy on the other side last year, when she developed a cough which did not resolve and unfortunately on a scan was found to have lung metastases.

She had had a course of chemotherapy which had finished a month ago, but the lung metastases had not improved much so her oncologist discussed a trial of the new agent called a PARP inhibitor. This was not the usual kind of randomized trial, as the drug was being tested to see how effective it was rather than comparing against 'standard' treatment—Beth was told there is no real 'standard' treatment for her situation.

Beth entered the trial and was pleased to find she coped well with treatment – she had a week on the drug via a drip then 2 weeks off the drug. The lung metastases did indeed seem to shrink on the scans and her cough resolved. She is continuing on the trial for 3 months.

13

Advanced and recurrent breast cancer

⮕ Key Points

◆ Breast cancer that is locally advanced means large tumours over about 5cm or fixed to skin or chest wall.

◆ The commonest sites of distant metastases from a breast cancer are to bone, liver and lung.

◆ Locally advanced and metastatic breast cancer is usually treated with chemotherapy and/or hormonal therapy.

◆ Treatment for metastatic breast cancer aims to control symptoms and maintain the best possible quality of life.

Breast cancer that presents at an advanced stage

Early and metastatic breast cancer

Most women who develop breast cancer— in fact well over 90%— will have what is called early breast cancer. This means the cancer is confined to the breast and sometimes also the lymph nodes under the arm (the axilla), but has not spread to other parts of the body. Very occasionally when a woman first finds the cancer in her breast, it will already have spread elsewhere in the body—*metastatic* disease. This usually only happens if the breast cancer is large at presentation and has already spread to the lymph nodes. Sometimes clues to this spread are symptoms such as bone pain, jaundice or shortness of breath. However, usually it is only found when the woman has tests on the rest of the body to look for disease. Because it is so unusual for early breast cancer to spread (if the disease in the breast is small and is not in the lymph nodes) women with these early cancers are not routinely screened for metastases to other sites in the body.

Sometimes this metastatic cancer will occur without there even being an obvious cancer in the breast and will present with, for example, bone pain.

Because the commonest sites of metastasis are to bones, lungs and the liver, the tests to look for these will usually include blood tests, a bone scan, and CT scans of the chest and abdomen or whole body MRI (or a chest X-ray and liver ultrasound). There are some breast cancer markers which are measured by blood tests and can be useful for some women. PET scans are not often useful in breast cancer. These are also the tests used to monitor metastatic disease and its response to treatment.

If a suspected tumour is seen at a distant site in the body it may be biopsied, usually by needle biopsy, to confirm it is cancer. However, in some areas of the body this is not possible so the diagnosis rests on the imaging appearance.

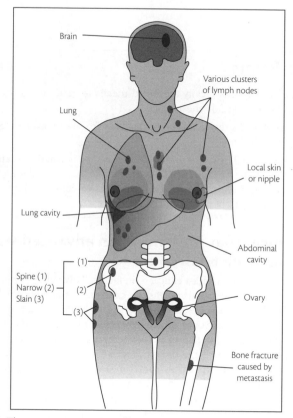

Figure 13.1 The most common sites of breast cancer metastasis.

Women who are first found to have cancer in the breast that has already spread elsewhere in the body are not usually offered surgery to the breast, but instead are treated with chemotherapy or hormonal therapy. However, there is sometimes value in removing the cancer in the breast so it does not cause unpleasant symptoms. There is also some suggestion that this may improve overall outcomes by decreasing the total amount of tumour in the body, and so allowing treatments such as chemotherapy to work better.

> ### Staging tests for the spread of breast cancer include:
>
> ◆ Blood tests
> ◆ Bone scan
> ◆ CT scan or
> ◆ Chest X-ray and ultrasound

Locally advanced breast cancer

Another type of advanced cancer is locally advanced breast cancer. This means disease which is in the breast and/or lymph nodes, but is very large (over 5 centimetres), fixed to the skin or the underlying chest wall muscles or actually causing ulceration of the skin or nipple. This kind of cancer is more likely to be associated with distant metastases so these women will have tests of the rest of their body. A special kind of advanced breast cancer is called inflammatory breast cancer. This can look almost like an infection of the breast—the breast is red, often hot and the skin thickened and puckered—called peau d'orange (or orange peel). This change is due to cancer cells permeating the tiny vessels under the skin and blocking the lymphatic drainage of the breast.

Locally advanced breast cancers are usually treated with chemotherapy (neo-adjuvant chemotherapy) prior to surgery and radiotherapy. In some cases a surgeon may feel it is not possible to remove the whole tumour in the first instance (for example inflammatory breast cancer) so the role of this up-front chemotherapy is to make mastectomy possible. In other cases the cancer would be amenable to mastectomy when the patient first presents but the aim of chemotherapy is to shrink the tumour to perhaps allow for lumpectomy.

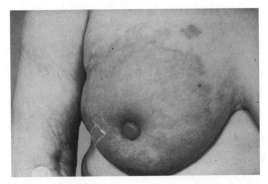

Figure 13.2 Inflammatory breast cancer.

Recurrent breast cancer

Although breast cancer treatment is increasingly successful for the majority of women, for some the disease will come back. This can be in the breast or chest wall skin, after mastectomy, and can be picked up either by the woman herself, an examining doctor or nurse or on her routine follow-up mammogram. A recurrence in the breast or on the chest wall is typically a hard nodule just under the skin, often close to the scar of the previous operation.

Recurrence can also be to other sites in the body. The commonest is to bones—which can cause either bone pain or anaemia if the bone marrow is involved and not producing red blood cells. Other sites include the liver (which can result in liver malfunction and jaundice), the lungs (which can cause a cough and short-ness of breath) and the brain (resulting in headaches or even faints or fits).

Table 13.1 Sites and symptoms of breast cancer metastases

Site	Symptom
Local recurrence	Nodule often near scar
Bone	Pain, fracture or anaemia
Liver	Abdominal pain and bloating or jaundice
Lungs	Cough or shortness of breath
Brain	Headaches or faints

The chance of breast cancer recurring will depend on the stage of the cancer when it is first diagnosed (see Chapter 6). With treatment most breast cancers will not recur.

It is important to realise that everyone gets symptoms such as bone ache from time to time and in a woman who has had breast cancer these are usually *not* due to cancer recurrence. However, any persisting symptoms should be reported to a doctor.

Prognosis of advanced breast cancer

The chance of cure for a woman with any type of advanced breast cancer—whether it is locally advanced in the breast or metastatic—is much worse than for women with early disease.

Breast cancer that has spread to other sites of the body is rarely curable. This means it is likely that one day this will be the cause of the woman's death. The aim of treatment is therefore to control the disease for as long as possible and ensure the best quality of life.

In women with bone metastases this control of disease can last for many years—even decades. If the breast cancer has spread to other organs such as the liver or lungs the prognosis is not as good and most women will lose their lives to the cancer within a few years—although there are some women who live (and live very well) with metastatic breast cancer for over 10 years. Another important indicator of poor outlook is the speed with which a breast cancer returns after initial treatment.

Locally advanced breast cancer, and cancer that recurs in the breast only, is a much more mixed bag of diseases. It is certainly still potentially curable, although some locally advanced cancers, and in particular inflammatory cancers, often behave in an aggressive way and although they may be controlled locally for a time, will spread to other organs within a few years. The number of women who remain cancer-free with locally advanced disease is about half that of those with early disease.

The newer treatments for breast cancer mean anything we say about the outcomes of disease today may not be accurate in a year or two—exciting developments in targeted drugs (see Chapter 12) and even the long-term results for the newer drugs we are currently using, such as Herceptin, are not yet known, but are likely to mean women can live much longer with metastatic disease, and hopefully retain a good quality of life.

Controlling disease in the breast, on the chest wall and in the axilla

Surgery is the best form of controlling breast cancer in the breast and axilla, if it is possible. If, after breast-conservation surgery, the cancer returns in the breast or the axilla, a mastectomy is needed—it is very difficult to give radiotherapy twice to the same area. It may be possible to remove nodules of cancer from the chest wall if they are small and very localized. If the woman has not had previous radiotherapy this may be a good option.

Drug treatments such as hormone therapies and chemotherapy can also be used to treat the recurrent cancer in the breast or chest wall.

Controlling metastatic breast cancer

Treatments aimed at controlling metastatic disease aim to improve length and quality of a woman's life but generally are not aimed at curing the breast cancer. It is important that any treatments used do not cause worse side-effects than the symptoms they are aiming to treat. Treating metastatic breast cancer should be a team effort—it usually involves the oncologist, the general practitioner and often other medical and supportive care people, as well as, of course, the woman and her family.

Drugs for advanced disease

Like early breast cancer, the drugs used for advanced disease are hormone therapy if the cancer is hormone-responsive, chemotherapy, and targeted therapies such as Herceptin, if the cancer is responsive to these. The receptor 'status' or responsiveness or recurrent breast cancer is usually the same as that of the tumour when it was first diagnosed.

The type of drug used for recurrent breast cancer will vary considerably from patient to patient and will depend on what drugs the woman has received before, what sort of response she had to those drugs, and to an extent the site and amount of recurrent cancer.

Bone metastases often respond very well to hormone drugs such as Tamoxifen and aromatase inhibitors or in pre-menopausal women to stopping ovarian function. There are other kinds of hormone agents (for example fulvestrant and megace) which can be used one after another, although on the whole, the introduction of each new agent is somewhat less effective than the last.

Disease in the liver and lungs usually requires chemotherapy. The type of chemotherapy will depend on what a woman has had before and is often a complex decision with the medical oncologist. Herceptin does not get into the brain, but is very useful in other sites of disease if the tumour is one of the 15% or so that are responsive to it.

Many women with advanced disease will be offered treatment in a clinical trial. This is because it is in advanced disease that new agents are first tried out, and if a woman has had many of the conventional drugs and the disease still persists, she may get benefit from some of these drugs.

Another common drug used for patients with advanced disease is a bisphosphonate—these are drugs such as aledronate, clodronate and pamidronate which help in bone metastases by keeping calcium levels normal and helping heal the diseased bone.

Many women with advanced cancer will also require pain relief (for example for bone pain), and help with other symptoms. Some of this is discussed below under Palliative care.

Drugs used in metastatic disease include:

- Hormone therapy such as Tamoxifen, aromatase inhibitors, progesterone drugs (such as megace), fulvestrant, ovarian suppression
- Chemotherapy
- Targeted treatments such as Herceptin
- Bisphosphonates for bone metastasis
- Pain relief

Other treatments for advanced disease

Radiotherapy is commonly used to treat bone metastases, and is usually a short course (one to two weeks) to the painful area such as the back or hip.

Surgery can occasionally be used for metastases to sites such as the liver, if it is thought the disease is not widespread throughout the body, and if the surgery is going to improve the patients' quality of life.

Many women turn to complementary and alternative treatments during the advanced stage of their disease. Many complementary therapies can be very helpful in alleviating symptoms—these are covered in Chapter 14.

> It is important that women look closely at some of the complementary and alternative therapies on offer, particularly those that come at a high financial cost, as there may be little or no benefit and some can even do more harm than good.

Psychosocial issues and advanced breast cancer

Being diagnosed with recurrent breast cancer can be more devastating even than the original diagnosis. This applies not just to the woman but to her family. Younger women often suffer most acutely from this, particularly those with dependent children.

As discussed in Chapter 14, women with advanced breast cancer are more likely to develop depression and other psychological issues. The physical problems such as discomfort, pain, tiredness, poor appetite, stomach problems, sexual problems and lymphoedema that can be associated with advanced disease may make psychological functioning worse. This can be exacerbated by a woman not being able to function normally. Having to give up work, day-to-day activities or social activities and having poor mobility will affect quality of life. It is important women discuss these with their health care team as they can be addressed.

A good diet, with advice if needed from a dietician, and physical activity if it can be tolerated, will also help many symptoms. Addressing practical issues is also important—getting help around the house, getting financial advice and legal advice about your will.

Palliative care

Palliative care means controlling patients' symptoms in association with optimising their emotional, social and spiritual well-being. Many people fear the idea of palliative care as they feel it is 'giving up treatment'. In fact it is far from this—it may involve all sorts of active treatments and is aimed at making a person live the best quality of life they can for as long as they can, even if they cannot be cured of their cancer.

> Palliative care is aimed at making a person live the best quality of life they can for as long as they can, even if they cannot be cured of their cancer.

Palliative care is practised by specialist palliative care physicians as well as specialist nurses and GPs. Many oncologists will be very involved in this side of treatment and all will work closely with palliative care colleagues.

Palliative care can mean advice in an outpatient setting, home visits by a specialist team or GP, or sometimes being cared for in a hospice or palliative care ward in a hospital. It is worth establishing contact early with a palliative care team as they can help address all sorts of problems a patient with advanced cancer may have, and are the most experienced of all health professionals at this. They can plan ahead and not just respond to problems or crises as they arise.

The palliative care team can also support the family of a person with advanced cancer, and offer help during bereavement. Planning for the end of life with dignity and without pain or other debilitating symptoms is a vital part of coping with advanced breast cancer.

14

Coping with breast cancer

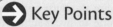

Key Points

- Up to a third of women suffer anxiety and/or depression in the year after breast cancer diagnosis.

- Depression is more likely to occur in women with a history of depression, in very young women, in those who lack social support and in women with advanced disease.

- There are good treatments for depression so a woman should seek medical help.

- There are many avenues for support for women with breast cancer including the treating team, the GP and community support groups.

- Complementary therapies can help women cope with some of the effects of breast cancer and good web-based information on many of these is available.

How breast cancer can affect a woman and her family

Breast cancer will affect well over a million women globally each year, and for each of these women, her family, her friends and her colleagues there will be a different set of experiences and range of effects. However, most will experience not only the physical effects of cancer and its treatment but psychological and emotional challenges as well as practical ones. This chapter outlines what some of these are—and although many may be 'normal' effects for women and their families in this situation, women may need help and strategies to manage these.

It is possible to list some of the effects of breast cancer—the physical consequences of surgery and radiotherapy, the side-effects of chemotherapy, shock of diagnosis and concerns about one's survival, anger, isolation and depression that may follow diagnosis and treatment, and loss of libido and sexual feelings, change in employment and financial worries. These are just some issues—they are often interconnected and it is a bit artificial to try to separate them. However, we will try to address some of the common problems women face when coping with breast cancer and suggest ways they may alleviate these.

A person reading this book has already taken a first step in improving their ability to cope with breast cancer—information and understanding the disease *will* help.

Psychological issues

Anxiety and depression are common side-effects of cancer and its treatment—up to a third of women will experience significant symptoms either around diagnosis or in the few years following it. However, these are also fairly common conditions in people without cancer—in fact nearly one in five adults will experience depression or severe anxiety at some point in their lives. So women with breast cancer may already have had this problem—and the cancer can certainly cause it to recur or get worse.

Some women are more at risk than others of developing psychological problems—those with a past history of these, those who are socially isolated or have limited support networks of family and friends, younger women and those with more advanced disease and those suffering chronic pain.

Symptoms of anxiety include poor concentration, poor sleep and persisting feelings of worry and unrest. Some women will experience panic attacks. These should be discussed with the health care team and can be helped by relaxation and other behaviour therapies and sometimes by anti-anxiety medication.

Table 14.1 Depression: common symptoms and management strategies

Symptoms of depression	Managing depression
Persistent low mood	Discuss with family
Sleep disturbances	Discuss with health care practitioner
Fatigue	Referral to psychologist
Loss of interest in usually enjoyable activities	Contact with support groups
	Consider antidepressant medication

Symptoms of depression include persistent low mood, loss of interest in things which normally were enjoyable, poor sleep, extreme fatigue and sometimes loss of appetite. Of course many of these things are 'normal' during cancer treatment, but if they are disrupting quality of life, seeking help can be useful. Sometimes just discussing the problems, with a GP, the breast nurse or the specialist, can lead to coping strategies, but many women find benefit from referral to a psychologist. Some will benefit from antidepressant medication.

Body image and sexuality

All the treatments for breast cancer can affect how your body looks and feels and how you feel about it. The effects of surgery are most obvious but radiotherapy can also lead to tenderness and an uncomfortable breast. Chemotherapy may lead to hair loss, fatigue, nausea, and early menopause in younger women, and some hormonal treatments may cause vaginal dryness. All of these can lead to a lower libido and lack of interest in sex.

There are some things you may do to help with this: talking to your partner and finding ways to adapt to the situation will help. Lubricants and vaginal moisturisers can help with the dryness—your health care team can advise on these. Your health care team can also refer you to a specialist relationship or sex counsellor which may help you and your partner.

Support available

Most people will have some resources of their own to cope with the psychological consequences of cancer—however for many these will be stretched and asking for emotional, informational and practical help from health care professionals will help many women cope better. In fact counselling is proven to help relieve some of the distress women feel after breast cancer, and leads to better quality of life.

A woman's own support network

Discussing your feelings with family and friends, and asking for help when needed, will not only help you, but will allow those around you to express their feelings and feel of some practical use. There will inevitably be a few friends who are not supportive during your cancer—this may be because they find it difficult to cope with their own fears and feelings of the disease.

Breast nurses

Most public hospitals and increasing numbers of private ones will have trained breast nurses as part of the team looking after women with breast cancer. The role of a breast nurse is wide-ranging (Chapter 7 discusses this further) but they are often the best source of how to access information, how to get psychological, financial and practical help and are also well trained in helping women cope with many of the strains of diagnosis and treatment. Most women will meet the breast nurse at the beginning of their breast cancer journey. However, psychological problems can occur at any time—often after active treatment has finished. Most breast nurses are happy to help and direct a patient to appropriate support at any time, so contacting them even after active treatment finishes is OK.

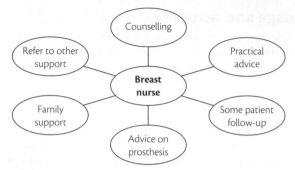

Figure 14.1 The role of the breast nurse.

Counselling

Psychological counselling may involve just talking to a trained professional counsellor, but can include treatments such as relaxation therapy, educational and behavioural treatments and sometimes referral for medications. You can ask any member of the treatment team or your GP for referral to a psychologist or counsellor, and this is usually covered by health insurance.

General practitioner

Having a regular GP may be the most important part of your overall health care. They can be a sounding board for your treatment decisions but also look after your health generally and be involved in the follow-up care after cancer. They are an excellent place to start when discussing your emotional and psychological concerns.

Peer support

There are many organizations and individual groups who have various forms of support that breast cancer patients can access. This may include meeting up individually with another woman who has experienced breast cancer, groups of breast cancer survivors, and groups who provide information and resources to women who have had breast cancer. A good example of this is the Breast Cancer Network Australia's 'My Journey Kit'. Your treatment team or local cancer organization should be able to provide information on these.

Support for your partner

The partner of a woman with breast cancer can feel frustrated that the situation is not in their control, worried about how they may feel about their partners body changes, have difficulty coping with the emotional problems both they and their partner face and feel isolated with no one to discuss their own feelings with. Many may feel guilty and worried about finances, but feel it is not the time to discuss these issues with their partner who is going through treatment.

It is normal for a partner to feel all these things, and there are things that can help.

Getting information about treatments and support, getting organized, being practical and asking for help from others if needed are all good strategies. Making time to spend with each other, even having fun in such a situation, can both help maintain and even improve a relationship, as can opening good lines of communication.

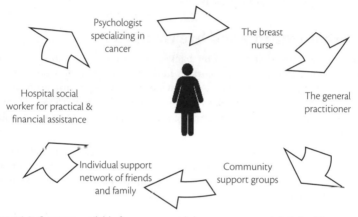

Figure 14.2 Support available for women with breast cancer and their families.

Telling children about breast cancer

Most children will realise even without being told that there is something wrong, so talking to them is important. Like all of us, children find it easier to cope with things if they know the nature of what they are facing. Finding out about their concerns is important and may help explain what can seem like their bad behaviour.

Very young children are scared they will be abandoned but may only be able to express this by becoming clinging. It is important they know it is not their fault mum has cancer. Older children and teenagers can find it hard to express themselves. Again information on the cancer and how it will impact on the family will help them face the situation. Explaining that the experience they are going through is not unique to them and exploring their feeling will help. Letting them be part of the support for their family and allowing them to be sad or angry is OK. They may find it useful to talk to someone—there are now good support groups for children of parents with cancer. Sometimes a visit to a counsellor can help.

Recommended further reading

📕 **Helping Your Children Cope with Your Cancer: A Guide for Parents and Families** by Peter Van Dernoot, (2002). Hatherleigh Press, New York, New York. ISBN: 1-57826-105-8.

📕 **Helping Children Cope with the Loss of a Loved One, A Guide for Grownups** by William C. Kroen, (1996). Free Spirit Publishing, Minneapolis, MN. ISBN: 1-57542-000-7.

Different cultures and breast cancer

Breast cancer affects women of all backgrounds. In some cultures it is more difficult to talk about than in others. A huge barrier for some women is when English is not their first language—most hospitals can provide an interpreter service which may be better than relying on family for translation. The opportunity to discuss the disease and treatment with a member of one's own cultural group can be invaluable.

All consultations with health care staff are confidential, and they have the obligation to respect patients' cultural and spiritual beliefs. If it is important that a woman be treated by a female health professional this should be made clear and the staff will do their utmost to help.

Getting breast cancer is not the fault of anyone and women need not feel guilty about it.

Practical needs

Apart from the emotional and physical cost of cancer, the diagnosis can bring a number of practical problems. Having to give up work, travel for treatment, childcare, paying for treatment (in particular the cost of breast reconstruction or drug treatments may be considerable in some areas) and paying for things such as wigs, prostheses and physiotherapy all bring a financial burden. The hospital social worker is well placed to advise on financial issues and help, and the breast nurse can also advise. Some local cancer organizations offer practical and financial help.

Grief

Grief is a common emotion after breast cancer—for the woman and her family. She may be grieving for the loss of her breast or body image, for her femininity, for her survival. This is a natural process which is part of coming to terms with the new reality, but in fact is necessary to move on with life. There may be stages of grief—shock, denial, anger, adjustment and finally acceptance—and everyone experiences these differently. If it becomes impossible to cope with these feelings and they seem to last forever it is worth seeking counselling.

Complementary therapy

These are treatments which are used along with medical and drug treatments to help manage symptoms and improve well-being. They are not cancer treatments per se. Alternative therapy is what is usually meant when therapies are used instead of conventional medical treatment. There are many examples of complementary therapies which range from group therapy such as yoga to touch-based techniques such as reiki. Many cancer treatment centres will now have direct access to these treatments, whether from individual practitioners or in an integrated centre. Many are also rebatable through health insurance schemes. There are some well regarded websites which give information on these therapies. Many cancer organizations have lists of local services.

📄 Case study

Margaret is a 55-year-old secretary who has been diagnosed with widespread DCIS in her left breast through a screening mammogram. She undergoes a mastectomy and does not need any further treatment. Her treatment team and her family are delighted she is 'cured' of her cancer and she is discharged from active treatment, only needing follow-up every six months.

However, over the course of the next few months Margaret cannot shake off feelings of sadness and concern. She is constantly worried the cancer will come back in the other breast, or may spread and kill her (even though she has been reassured it is pre-invasive and thus cannot spread). She feels ashamed of her mastectomy and takes to wearing covering clothes—she will not let her husband see her body and has lost all interest in sex. Yet she cannot talk to her husband about it as it seems almost trivial as everyone else seemed so delighted she was cured.

Gradually Margaret finds it harder and harder to get up for work each day, and uses the excuse of early retirement to stop altogether. She cannot sleep at night and feels tired and flat all day.

Her husband recognizes this but finds it hard to discuss with her—he does miss having sex but would not push her to and stops touching her as he feels this just upsets her.

At her 6 month follow-up visit the breast nurses recognise there are some problems and encourage both Margaret and her husband to go for some counselling. Margaret and her husband discuss with the counsellor about how she is feeling and together they are able to learn to overcome some of the issues. A short course of anti-depressants from the GP is suggested but in fact Margaret finds that a regular exercise programme put on by a local breast cancer support group, understanding her depression and learning to communicate with her husband help her not only overcome her depression but start to enjoy physical contact with her husband again.

15

Special circumstances

⮕ Key Points

◆ Around 1 in 20 women who develop breast cancer under the age of 45 years will develop it during pregnancy or breastfeeding.

◆ Fertility can be affected by cancer treatment and if this is of concern to a woman she should discuss it with a specialist.

◆ Male breast cancer is rare but does occur and can be related to a family history of the disease.

◆ Breast cancer poses a number of extra burdens for very young women including those of more radical treatments, body image, relationship and psychological issues, issues relating to early menopause and the effects of the diagnosis on young children.

◆ Breast cancer commonly affects elderly women and the risks of treatments need to be weighed up against the benefits to keep a woman healthy and with a good quality of life.

This chapter touches on some of the more unusual circumstances in which breast cancer affects people. These will often require a highly specialized and experienced team to give the patient and family the best possible information and treatment to ensure the best outcome.

Breast cancer and pregnancy

Whilst breast cancer is fortunately a very rare event in pregnant and breastfeeding women, it does occur occasionally—around 5% of breast cancers in women under 45 years occur at this time. This stresses the need for any woman to have a breast symptom thoroughly checked out—a lump which comes up during pregnancy and persists over a few weeks should be reported to a doctor and investigated. The tests done during pregnancy are the same as in any other woman (see Chapter 5)—even mammograms can be safely carried out with proper shielding of the unborn baby.

If a woman is diagnosed during pregnancy this is likely to be a pretty devastating event for her and her family, and unusual enough that it warrants care by a highly specialized team. Unless the woman is in the very early stages of pregnancy there is no good reason to terminate the pregnancy unless this is her wish. Surgery can be performed during pregnancy but radiotherapy cannot, so surgery is often by mastectomy unless it can wait until after delivery of the baby. Chemotherapy can safely be given after the first trimester (12 weeks) of pregnancy, although hormonal agents such as Tamoxifen should wait until after delivery.

If breast cancer is found during breastfeeding, women are usually advised to stop feeding as any chemotherapy can travel through the milk to the baby. It is not possible to feed from a breast that has had radiotherapy.

Treatments during pregnancy and lactation

Surgery:

◆ Usually mastectomy is recommended

Radiotherapy:

◆ Avoided during pregnancy

◆ Can be safely given after delivery

Chemotherapy:

◆ Can be given during pregnancy after the first trimester

◆ Women should not breastfeed during chemotherapy

Tamoxifen:

◆ Should be avoided when pregnant

Unfortunately many of the treatments used in breast cancer will lower fertility and conceiving after breast cancer is not very common—in fact less than half the number of women one would expect to get pregnant in a healthy population do so after cancer. However, if a woman and her partner are prepared to accept that her cancer can come back and interfere with her ability to care for a child, and she is not on any treatment, there is no good reason a woman cannot go on to have children after breast cancer if she is able to.

A subsequent pregnancy does not increase the chance of cancer recurrence and previous cancer treatment does not affect the baby.

Generally *in vitro* fertilization (IVF) is not recommended in women who have had breast cancer as the high doses of hormones potentially may increase recurrence risk, although we do not have much information on this.

Fertility after breast cancer

Cancer treatments can affect fertility. The older a woman is, the more likely chemotherapy is to damage her ovaries—on average chemotherapy will 'age' the ovaries by 10 years. Some chemotherapy agents are more toxic than others on the ovaries and this should be discussed with the oncologist.

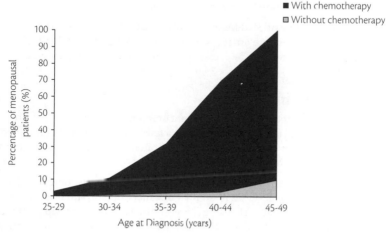

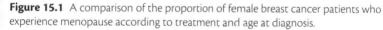

Figure 15.1 A comparison of the proportion of female breast cancer patients who experience menopause according to treatment and age at diagnosis.

There are some strategies to overcome this and any young woman facing chemotherapy who is concerned about future fertility should have the opportunity to discuss this with a specialist gynaecologist.

Some options which may be available to preserve potential fertility include:

♦ Embryo cryopreservation (freezing) which is suitable for women with a partner but does require a cycle of IVF to collect the eggs—this can delay cancer treatment and its safety is not known. Delaying this until after chemotherapy will dramatically reduce its chance of success.

♦ For women without a partner egg freezing is possible but the pregnancy rate is very low after this procedure and again it requires a cycle of IVF to collect the eggs.

♦ For those who do not wish to undertake IVF or to delay treatment, ovarian tissue freezing which can later be transplanted back into the woman may be an option. However, only two live human births worldwide have been reported following this procedure.

♦ Temporarily shutting down the ovaries during chemotherapy may protect them. This can be done with injections of drugs such as goserelin (Zoladex). It is still not proven if this will help maintain fertility.

♦ IVF with donor eggs can be considered for couples when the woman goes into early menopause from cancer treatment. Success rates are relatively high but practical and psychological issues associated with finding a suitable donor must be considered and the safety of IVF is still unknown.

♦ Having a surrogate mother carry a pregnancy offers the advantage of avoiding oestrogen stimulation after cancer.

♦ Adoption remains a possibility for some couples.

To add to these complexities, different countries have different laws and regulations relating to infertility treatment, surrogacy and adoption, and there are also the ethical dilemmas relating to social acceptance and religious, cultural, and spiritual beliefs.

Breast cancer in men

Breast cancer can occur in men but is uncommon—less than 1% of breast cancers are in men and in most countries only a few hundred a year are diagnosed. It usually affects older men and occurs more often in families which carry a high risk gene—the *BRCA 2* gene.

As breast cancer is often seen as a 'woman's cancer' some men find it difficult or embarrassing talking about it. A number of cancer organizations around the world are recognizing that men also get breast cancer and are providing information and help specifically aimed at men: see the National Breast and Ovarian Cancer Centre (NBOCC) website.

Breast cancer in men usually presents as a lump in the tissue behind the nipple or lumps under the arm—the lymph nodes. The investigation is the same as for women (see Chapter 5) and treatments are also largely the same—surgery, radiotherapy and hormone or chemotherapy where appropriate.

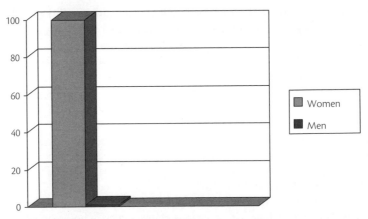

Figure 15.2 Comparison breast cancer rates in men and women.

Second cancers

Breast cancer can recur and the chance of this happening will depend on the prognostic features of the cancer (see Chapter 6). A woman can also get a second breast cancer in either the treated breast or the other side. In fact women who have had one breast cancer are about twice as likely to get another. So it is very important to undergo regular—usually annual—screening with examination and mammograms to pick up any further disease very early.

We know that five years of a hormone drug such as Tamoxifen or an aromatase inhibitor will reduce the chance of a second breast cancer by 50%. There are a number of studies going on to see if taking these drugs even longer term may protect more. However, a few women are not happy accepting this risk and opt to undergo bilateral mastectomy.

Women who carry a high risk gene for breast cancer are unfortunately even more likely to get another cancer, and often wish to consider prophylactic surgery. This may be especially relevant in this group of women as cancers associated with these genes can be quite rapidly growing and come up between screens.

Breast cancer in very young women

Breast cancer does not occur often in very young women. If we define very young as under 40, less than 6% of breast cancers will occur in this age group. Unfortunately cancers seem to be diagnosed when larger and can be more aggressive in very young women, leading to a lower chance of cure for women in their thirties. Around 85% will be alive five years after diagnosis, compared to over 90% in women over this age. This is slightly worse for women in their twenties at diagnosis.

Young women do have a particular set of problems, not least the fact that they often feel isolated and unique for having a disease like breast cancer at such a young age. Some of these issues are discussed below.

Risk factors for very young women

For many the first question they will have is 'why did I get cancer at this age?' Breast cancer in very young women is more likely to be due to an inheritable fault in one of the 'breast cancer genes' (see Chapter 2). This can be the case even if there is no, or only a fairly distant, family history of the disease. This should be discussed with the treatment team and it may be appropriate for a young woman to be referred to a family cancer clinic to discuss this further. They can arrange for genetic testing which may affect further treatment decisions as well as have consequences for other family members.

However, most young women (over 80%) with breast cancer do *not* carry one of the known cancer genes, and we really do not know the cause of cancer in these women.

Diagnosis in very young women

Screening using mammography is not useful in most very young women as the density of the breast tissue makes it hard to detect any abnormality. It is important that even young women are aware of how their breasts normally look and feel and how this can change with the menstrual cycle, and that they report any persisting changes to their doctor and get these adequately investigated.

> Most breast cancers will be found by the young woman herself (or her partner) as a lump.

Treatment of very young women

Although the same principles of treatment apply to women of all ages, there is some evidence that very young women may have a somewhat increased chance of local recurrence if they conserve the breast. This, along with the fact that tumours can be larger and more aggressive in young women, means they are more likely to have a mastectomy—and more likely to have reconstruction (see Chapter 8). However, young women are also more likely to suffer from psychological stresses and undoubtedly the need to lose a breast will contribute to this.

> Seeking good counselling and psychosocial support is extremely important.

Because most breast cancers are fairly aggressive in younger women, most will be encouraged to have chemotherapy. This can have effects on fertility, as discussed above, and may also lead to early menopause with all the problems associated with this (see Chapter 16).

Contraception

It is certainly important that a woman on active treatment such as chemotherapy or hormone therapy does not get pregnant during this treatment—even if her periods stop this is still possible. Finding the right contraception is essential. It is not recommended that women use the oral contraceptive pill or the depot implant/injection after breast cancer so alternative methods such as condoms need to be tried.

Relationships

Young women are more likely to have struggles regarding relationships after breast cancer—if a young woman is single just starting a new relationship can be hard—having a new partner see you for the first time with a mastectomy scar is a pretty daunting experience.

Women in a relationship also report more problems due to body image and loss of feelings of femininity, poor libido, loss of fertility, menopause symptoms, depression and just coping with the stresses of a busy life and cancer treatment.

> Good and open communication, counselling (including with the partner) and finding out as much as possible about the symptoms being experienced are important steps.

Children

Many women at this stage of life will have a young family, and coping with this whilst undergoing cancer treatment is a real challenge. Asking for help from family and friends (getting other mothers to do the school runs for instance), and getting in touch with agencies that can provide assistance will help.

Work and finances

Loss of income, loss of pension, and difficulties obtaining insurance or a mortgage are real problems facing some young women with breast cancer. This may be made worse if they have to pay for some of the treatment. Some local cancer organisations or the social work department at the hospital can help address these issues.

If a woman does need to take significant time off work (which most do) discussing the reason with the employer should lead them to be supportive, and contacting a union representative can also help.

Diet and exercise

A healthy diet and regular exercise are important for all women after breast cancer—regular exercise has been shown to improve the fatigue associated with treatment, improve mood and help depression, it may help menopause symptoms—and importantly it may even improve survival. There are a number of groups that organize specific programmes for women after cancer—a breast nurse will be able to advise what is available locally.

Needs of younger women with advanced disease

Younger women find it more difficult to make the transition from curative to non-curative treatment, and are more likely to suffer depression with advanced disease. Early consultation with the palliative care team can be useful to help address symptoms and find good ways to manage them.

> It is important to realise that even advanced disease is treatable and many women will live a very long time with a good quality of life even in the face of metastatic breast cancer.

Breast cancer in the elderly

Older women who develop breast cancer may also face particular challenges, mostly due to the fact that many will have a number of coexisting medical conditions, and may be more frail and so less able to tolerate some of the treatments for breast cancer. There is also evidence that chemotherapy may not be so effective in older women.

For any woman presenting with early breast cancer, surgery is the best option to control the disease in the breast. A higher proportion of elderly women choose mastectomy as this will usually mean that they can avoid radiotherapy—and many do not want the inconvenience of travelling for this daily for six weeks, or would find it difficult to lie in the position needed to carry out to the radiotherapy, or perhaps have a partner whom they have to care for.

If a patient is really not fit enough to undergo a general anaesthetic and surgery, and she had a tumour which is hormone-sensitive, then it is an option to treat with a hormone drug in the first instance (such as Tamoxifen or an aromatase inhibitor) and monitor the cancer to ensure it does not grow.

In making treatment choices, it is important elderly women and their families consider all the risks and benefits of treatment so they choose what is best for them—but it is also important to remember that humans are living longer and longer—for many of us 80 is no longer that elderly and a woman who survives to 80 and is fit is likely to survive at least another decade!

> **Keeping a woman healthy with the optimum quality of life should be the aim.**

16

Surviving after breast cancer

 Key Points

♦ Life after breast cancer can pose both physical and psychological challenges.

♦ Preventing lymphoedema with exercises and avoiding injury is important.

♦ Lymphoedema is treated with skin care, manual lymphatic drainage and compression garments.

♦ Menopause symptoms are common after breast cancer and most can be treated, usually with non-hormonal therapies.

After my very last radiation treatment for breast cancer, I lay on a cold steel table hairless, half-dressed and astonished by the tears streaming down my face. I thought I would feel happy about finally reaching the end of treatment, but instead I was sobbing. At the time I wasn't sure what emotions I was feeling. Looking back, I think I cried because this body had so bravely made it through 18 months of surgery, chemotherapy and radiation. Ironically, I also cried because I would not be coming back to that familiar table where I had been comforted and encouraged. Instead of joyous, I felt lonely, abandoned and terrified. This was the rocky beginning of cancer survivorship for me.

Elizabeth D. McKinley as quoted in Rowland *et al.*,
Journal of Clinical Oncology, 2006

The cancer has been treated, follow-up is a visit to the specialist only every 3 or 6 or even 12 months, and life is getting back to normal. But for many people the long term issues following both a diagnosis of cancer and the treatment for it remain a significant problem for years. For many it may, however, be a chance to re-evaluate life and priorities: cancer can strengthen a relationship and a family, be the kick start to actually getting healthier overall and may lead to other avenues in life.

In this final chapter we would like to touch on a few of the long-term issues that can affect breast cancer survivors—and the vast majority of women who develop breast cancer will be survivors. We will suggest strategies to manage some of the potential problems left after breast cancer and its treatment.

Lymphoedema

Fortunately lymphoedema is becoming a less common complication of breast cancer treatment. However, for the 10–20% of women who do develop this, it can be distressing and require significant treatment.

> Lymphoedema occurs in around 20% of women after axillary clearance but less than 2% after sentinel node biopsy.

Obviously, preventing lymphoedema or treating it very early are the best options— women having surgery or radiotherapy to the axilla should ideally be given education on this by a specialist physiotherapist or occupational therapist. Breast nurses will often be able to give advice.

Maintaining a healthy weight, physical activity and avoiding skin infections in the treated arm are important in prevention.

Early lymphoedema can often present not just as a swollen limb but as thickened tissues in the arm (or breast) and a persistent ache or heaviness. The mainstay of treatment is manual lymphatic drainage which is light and gentle massage which aims to drain the lymph out of the limb (or breast or chest wall). This can be taught to the woman herself or even her carers.

If the lymphoedema is more severe, compression sleeves and bandaging by a physiotherapist or occupational therapist can help. Keeping the arm elevated on a pillow at rest may be useful.

Exercise will definitely help both prevent and treat lymphoedema, and some exercises are based around a swimming programme. Ensuring the skin is well moisturised and avoiding infections are important will prevent worsening of the problem. Newer treatments which may help include low-level laser therapy, electrical stimulation and mechanical forms of massage. For a very few women surgery such as liposuction may be an option.

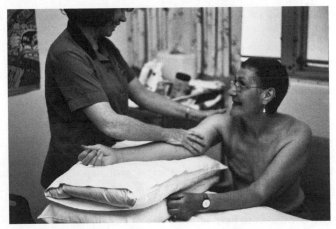

Figure 16.1 A patient receiving lymphoedema treatment.

Menopausal symptoms

Menopausal symptoms are extremely common sequelae of breast cancer treatments. They can lead to:

◆ Poor quality of life

◆ Psycho-sexual distress

◆ Cardiovascular problems such as increased rate of heart attacks and strokes

◆ Bone thinning or osteoporosis

Typical symptoms include:

◆ Hot flushes

◆ Night sweats

◆ Poor sleep

◆ A fall in sex drive

◆ Dry vagina

◆ Tiredness

◆ Mood changes

Of course many of these symptoms can occur after cancer treatment but are *not* related to menopause.

Menopausal symptoms can occur because the cancer treatment has caused an early menopause, or because a woman has had to come off her hormone replacement therapy (HRT) at diagnosis of cancer, or because these symptoms are a side-effect of the hormone drugs used to treat breast cancer—both Tamoxifen and the aromatase inhibitors.

Menopause symptoms can be quite mild and self-limiting, and many women are happy to undertake simple measures to control hot flushes such as wearing cotton clothing, dressing in layers so some can be removed, and avoiding triggers such as alcohol or spicy food. Weight loss, giving up smoking and exercise can also help.

Lifestyle strategies to help hot flushes:

♦ **Regular exercise**

♦ **Balanced diet—avoid spicy foods and excessive alcohol**

♦ **Avoid caffeine in food and drinks**

♦ **Wear clothes in layers**

Complementary treatments are popular but unfortunately there is little evidence they help menopausal symptoms, and a few can have side-effects—in particular progesterone-containing preparations (such as troches). Vitamin E may help decrease the number of hot flushes somewhat and acupuncture, relaxation therapy and biofeedback paced respiration may be useful for some women.

It is generally recommended that women should avoid HRT after breast cancer. The drug Tibilone (Livial) was thought to be safe but a recent study has shown a small increase in breast cancer recurrence in women taking this after breast cancer. However, there are a number of non-hormonal drugs such as Gabapentin and some of the antidepressants which will help hot flushes. Sometimes changing from one cancer hormone drug to another (such as from Tamoxifen to an aromatase inhibitor or vice versa) will also help.

Problems with vaginal dryness are particularly common in women on aromatase inhibitors. Vaginal moisturisers (such as Replens) and lubricants for use during sex can relieve this. Vaginal oestrogen creams are very good but there is a small question mark over their safety after breast cancer.

Question for the doctor: If I experience menopausal symptoms, can I be referred to a menopause specialist to discuss treatment for these?

The patient should discuss this option with her treating specialist and GP.

Bone health

Bones inevitably thin as we age, but if this becomes excessive it results in osteoporosis, and a much higher likelihood of fractures. In the elderly fractures can literally be life-threatening. Some people have an inherited risk of developing osteoporosis—if a woman's mother suffered this it is much more likely she may also.

Other things which increase the risk of osteoporosis include:

◆ Being very slender

◆ Smoking

◆ Excessive alcohol

◆ Not taking regular exercise

◆ Lack of calcium and vitamin D—the latter is needed to help absorb calcium and is formed by exposure to sunlight as well as the diet.

So getting 15 minutes or so a day of sunshine (weather permitting!) is good for you.

> It is important for all women as they get older (i.e. after the menopause) to take steps to keep their bones healthy—a good diet including 1200 mg daily of calcium in the diet or by supplements and around 1000 IU a day of vitamin D from fortified milk, eggs, fish or supplements, stopping smoking and weight-bearing exercises such as walking, dancing, jogging or tennis.

The female hormone oestrogen protects against osteoporosis so falls in this may contribute to thinning bones—this is what happens naturally after the menopause but is accelerated with an early menopause, such as that after breast cancer treatment, or with some of the breast cancer drugs such as aromatase inhibitors.

Women going on to an aromatase inhibitor, or those in whom thin bones may be an issue, should have a bone density test. Established osteoporosis can be treated with drugs called bisphosphonates. It is worth noting that Tamoxifen is protective of the bones and does not accelerate osteoporosis.

Fatigue

Fatigue is a common symptom during cancer treatment—patients report they have no energy and are tired all the time, despite resting. It may be due to the effects of surgery, radiotherapy and chemotherapy, as well as complex factors around feeling somewhat depressed, ceasing the usual routine including exercise, poor nutrition and poor sleep patterns. It can be combated with regular exercise, and facilitating sleep, sometimes short-term with medication.

However, fatigue can continue long term after active treatment has finished. It may not be possible to ascertain exactly why it is occurring but is worth discussing with your GP or specialist. Depression is commonly associated with fatigue and if present can be treated. Poor sleep and insomnia can be helped by a GP or even a specialist sleep clinic. The concept of 'sleep hygiene' or good sleep habits is important:

Sleep hygiene techniques

- Have a routine before bed such as a warm drink or a snack with tryptophan (such as a banana)
- Avoid alcohol and caffeine before bedtime
- Have a fixed bedtime
- Sleep in a quiet, dark, cool room with no distractions (no TV!)—the bedroom is for sleep and sex only
- Try relaxation techniques
- *Important*—sleep only when you are sleepy
- If you cannot fall asleep within about 20 minutes of going to bed, get up and do something boring!

Some people will have physical reasons for poor sleep such as sleep apnoea, which can cause frequent waking and which may need investigation and treatment. Lifestyle changes such as exercise and decreasing alcohol consumption will usually help fatigue, but it is important a doctor excludes other causes such as anaemia or an underactive thyroid.

Joint pains

Joint pains may be due to osteoarthritis or other joint conditions but are also a common side-effect of the aromatase inhibitor drugs, and can also sometimes occur after chemotherapy. Occasionally they can be due to the cancer spreading to the bones.

Joint pain due to the aromatase inhibitors will usually respond to the non-steroidal anti-inflammatory drugs (NSAIDs) you can buy over the counter at a chemist. Heat, massage, swimming and yoga can also help—it is useful to strengthen the muscles around a joint to help alleviate the pain.

Psychological issues

Uncertainty about the future and feelings of sadness or even depression can occur for long after the breast cancer has been successfully treated. These feelings may be particularly strong around the time of the regular check-up visit, but can be persistent and affect how a person functions and their quality of life.

It may be that the woman is only occasionally seeing a specialist for follow-up, and is probably no longer in contact with the breast nurse. However, these people should be made aware if there is a problem with depression, as they can discuss this, reassure any anxieties or even investigate any particular symptoms that may be of concern, or refer for counselling. Alternatively it is very appropriate to bring this up with a GP who will also be able to help.

Existential issues

Survivorship means maximizing quality of life by striving for optimal health in mind and body. This definition of health as total physical, mental and social well-being is the one given by the World Health Organization. Thus issues of our 'inner health' are vital to overall health.

> During treatment for breast cancer many women report that it is the fight to survive that is paramount—if they have younger children they will have a strong sense of purpose to care for them.

After active treatment it is thought that achieving peace of mind and a sense of purpose, learning to cope with negative thoughts and finding a 'new normal' are important parts of the healing process. This may take time and may mean the priorities that drove life before cancer need to be re-evaluated, and each person will have a different set of values to help them address this.

A survivorship plan

For each woman diagnosed with breast cancer each year there will be 10 others who have survived it and are getting on with their lives. The issues that are important to them include:

◆ Follow-up and surveillance for cancer recurrence or even a new breast cancer

◆ How to manage some of the symptoms discussed in this book such as menopausal symptoms and fertility concerns

◆ How to get their bodies back into good functioning order and cope with leftover problems of treatment such as pain and fatigue

◆ How to optimize their overall general health and lifestyle issues

◆ Ensuring their mental well-being is as good as it can be.

Many women do not receive the follow-up they would like from the specialists—consultations are infrequent, may be with different doctors each time, are often too brief to focus on all the issues they may wish to discuss. It is commonly reported that follow-up does not meet a woman's psychological needs. Some women will find many of these needs met by other health practitioners such as the GP, a nurse in a specialist clinic or a complementary therapist, but many would like a plan to help them achieve their own best health. The Lance

Armstrong Foundation in the United States has pioneered this approach and with the Institute of Medicine has come up with some sensible ideas.

A Survivorship Plan will include a record of treatment. This should include details of diagnostic tests, the pathology of the tumour, treatments received including when or if side-effects were experienced and details of who provided care.

Secondly, a Follow-up Care Plan can be designed for each individual. This should include:

◆ Recommended cancer screening including frequency of breast examination (and by whom), mammograms and any other regular tests.

◆ Information on long-term side-effects and how to seek help for these. This may include information on, for example, menopausal symptoms.

◆ How to look out for signs of recurrence or a new tumour. These may be local signs such as lumps in the skin of the chest wall, or persisting shortness of breath or bone pain which could indicate disease spread.

◆ Information on the effects of the cancer on psychosocial functioning such as possible effects on a relationship and sexual problems, with some suggestions on how to manage this.

◆ Financial consequences of cancer including work and insurance. This section may contain how to seek financial assistance or legal aid.

◆ Advice on a healthy lifestyle such as exercise, weight control, diet, prevention of osteoporosis and heart disease. How often to get regular check-ups of, for example, cholesterol, or how often to get Pap smears may be in this section.

◆ If appropriate, advice on genetic counselling and testing and surveillance. This may also include how relatives should be screened.

◆ Details on how to obtain referral to other specialists such as fertility experts, lymphoedema physiotherapists, counsellors, sex therapists.

◆ Details of support groups and a list of written and Internet-based resources.

If you do not have such a plan you could make one for yourself with the help of your health providers.

We have included a template for making a plan at the back of this book in the Appendix.

Acknowledgements and conclusion

We are privileged to have helped care for thousands of women and their families with breast cancer and it is from these women and their stories that we have drawn the inspiration for this book. We thank them.

We hope this book has given you some useful information. Information is power, and information is one of the best ways to cope with being diagnosed and treated for breast cancer. We hope you will look at some of the suggested websites and further reading materials, but most importantly we hope you recover, that you gain strength from your experiences and that you become one of the millions of women in the world who survive breast cancer and live your life how you want to, not how this disease tries to make you live it.

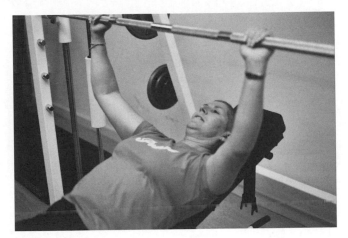

Figure 16.2 A survivor.

Appendix

Template for breast cancer survivorship plan

Survivor's name and date of birth:

This plan summarises information about your diagnosis, treatment, follow-up care, symptoms to watch out for and steps to staying healthy.

Cancer treatment summary

Cancer diagnosis

Date diagnosis

Stage at diagnosis

Pathology findings

Diagnostic tests and results

Treatment history

	Surgery	**Chemotherapy**	**Radiotherapy**
Date(s)			
Location			
Doctor			
(Name and telephone)			
Nurse			

	Hormonal therapy	**Other treatment**
Date(s)		
Location		
Doctor		
(Name and telephone)		
Nurse		

Risk of cancer recurrence

Patients should report the following symptoms and signs:

Recommended surveillance programme for recurrence or a new cancer includes

☐ Annual mammogram

☐ Check up by specialists in following schedule:

☐ Check up by GP every year

☐ Other tests as recommended by specialist:

☐ Other recommendations:

Potential late effects of treatment

Surgery

Radiotherapy

Chemotherapy

Hormonal therapy

Patients should report the following symptoms and signs:

Recommended surveillance for late effects includes:

Prevention strategies for late effects include:

The doctor who will monitor me for late effects is:

Identified concerns	**Referral to**	
☐Depression/anxiety	☐Psychology	☐Psychiatry
☐Fertility	☐Fertility expert	
☐Relationships	☐Counsellor	
☐Sexuality		
☐Family history	☐Genetic counsellor	
☐Menopause	☐Menopause expert	
☐Wellness	☐Exercise programme	☐Rehab
☐Employment	☐Social worker	
☐Lymphoedema	☐Physiotherapy or occupational therapy	
☐Other	☐Other	

Services to think about and where to access them:

Counselling

Genetic counselling

Home care

Dietician

Occupational therapy

Physiotherapy

Social worker

Pain clinic

Stress management programme

Complementary therapies

Support services

Glossary

Adjuvant treatment Therapy after the initial treatment, i.e. extra treatment. In breast cancer, this usually means chemotherapy, radiotherapy and/or hormonal therapy *after* surgery.

Anaemia Deficiency in red blood cells/low blood count. This means less oxygen-carrying capacity in the blood and earlier fatigue. Anaemic patients can look pale.

Anastrazole Anti-oestrogen tablet used daily in postmenopausal women with oestrogen-sensitive breast cancer.

Angiogenic Forming new blood vessels. Cancers are angiogenic; they build new blood supplies into the growing tumour mass.

Aromatase inhibitors Class of anti-oestrogen medications used in post meno-pausal women with oestrogen-sensitive breast cancer. They block the hormone aromatase which is responsible for synthesizing oestrogen outside of the ovaries. Includes Anastrazole, Letrozole and Exemestane.

Atypical ductal hyperplasia (ADH) Abnormal growth of breast milk duct cells which is a risk factor for, but does not constitute, breast cancer. Can be found nearby actual cancers and therefore, surgical biopsy is usually recommended.

Atypical lobular hyperplasia (ALH) Like ADH but occurs in the milk-producing lobules in the breast tissue. ALH also indicates an increased risk of cancer.

Axilla/axillary nodes Axilla is the area between the chest and the arm, bounded front and back by muscles. Within this tissue are lymph nodes or glands, which filter fluid from the arm and breast on its way back into the blood. Cancer can spread along these lymphatic routes.

Axillary clearance Surgical removal of lymphatic tissue from the axilla.

Benign Not cancerous.

Biopsy Examination of a piece of tissue removed from the body in order to look for the presence and extent of disease. Biopsies can be taken via needle with the patient awake (see **Core biopsy** and **Fine-needle aspiration**) or at surgery: see **Surgical biopsy**.

Bone scan Type of scan assessing the bones for disease such as cancer spread.

BRCA1/2 Breast cancer genes. These genes run in families and carry a high risk of breast, ovarian and sometimes, other cancers.

Breast-conserving therapy (BCT) A combination of surgery +/– radiotherapy in which the breast is preserved. An alternative to mastectomy for smaller cancers.

Breast reconstruction Surgical construction of a new breast after mastectomy using various combinations of other body tissues and/or implants. Can be done at the time of mastectomy (immediate) or after treatment is concluded (delayed).

Calcification The deposition of calcium into tissues. In the breast, this can be a marker of cancerous change and shows up as white dots on mammogram.

Carcinoma Cancer arising from the skin or lining of internal organs. Breast carcinoma arises from the cells lining the milk-producing lobules and/or ducts.

Chemotherapy Also known as cytotoxic therapy. The treatment of disease via chemical substances (drugs) that kill cells.

Clinical trial Research comparing the effects of different treatments or of treatment versus no treatment in patients with a similar disease.

Complementary therapy Treatments which are used along with medical and drug treatments to help manage symptoms and improve well-being.

Core biopsy Needle biopsy in which a small piece of tissue can be removed from the patient. Usually done awake, under local anaesthetic and can be guided by ultrasound or X-ray as required.

CT scan Scan using multiple X-rays reconstructed on computer to create representative images of various cross-sections ('slices') of the body.

Disease-free survival The period for which a patient is free of cancer after treatment.

Ductal carcinoma *in situ* (DCIS) Breast cancer arising from duct cells, which is still confined within the duct system. A pre-invasive breast cancer.

Embryo cryopreservation Removal and freezing of embryos (fertilized eggs) in order for later re-implantation into the uterus with the aim of pregnancy.

ER See **Oestrogen receptor**.

Erythema Inflammation of the skin and other shallow tissues, showing up as redness and swelling. May be in response to injury, infection or other irritation.

Familial breast cancer Breast cancer appearing in multiple family members—presumed secondary to a transmitted breast cancer gene.

Fibroadenoma Benign breast tumour made up of glandular and fibrous tissue. Typically occurs in younger women and is not a risk factor for cancer.

Fine-needle aspiration (FNA) Technique to sample cells and/or fluid from a cyst or solid mass via a thin needle. Usually done with the patient awake, with or without ultrasound guidance.

Genes Hereditary material that provides instructions for the body on how to build all cells and tissues. Can carry various characteristics through families.

Gene mutations Abnormalities in a gene, which may be passed on from parent to offspring or may be spontaneously occurring. Can lead to cells and tissues growing or functioning abnormally, manifesting as cancer or other disease.

Gonadotrophin-releasing hormone (GnRH) analogues Drugs which trick the pituitary gland into reducing production of luteinizing hormone (LH), which is required by the ovaries to drive oestrogen production. This puts the ovaries to 'sleep' creating a reversible menopause. Includes: Goserelin and Tryptorelin.

Grade A way of classifying cancers according to their appearance. Low-grade cancers have a lower risk of recurrence as opposed to high-grade cancers. Breast cancers are typically graded from 1 (low) to 3 (high).

Her2 Also known as cErbB-2. Stands for human epidermal growth factor receptor and is overactive in ~20% of breast cancers. The target of newer drugs like Herceptin.

Herceptin Also known as Trastuzumab. A newer type of therapy, which is very effective against **Her2**-positive cancers.

Histology Microscopic analysis of tissues.

Hookwire localization Technique of placing a wire into the breast under X-ray or ultrasound guidance to help the surgeon find **impalpable** lesions.

Hormone receptor A molecule in the breast cancer cell that is 'switched on' by the attachment of oestrogen or progesterone and may facilitate further growth/multiplication.

Hormone replacement therapy (HRT) Oestrogen and/or progesterone given to reduce the effects of menopause.

Hormonal therapy Anti-oestrogen and/or progesterone treatments used in hormone sensitive breast cancers.

Impalpable Undetectable by touch alone.

Imprint cytology A laboratory technique for rapid microscopic assessment of surgical and other tissue specimens.

Inflammatory cancer A type of locally advanced breast cancer that presents with a red, warm and swollen breast often with **peau d'orange**.

In situ In its original place. With regard to cancer, this indicates pre-invasive change—see **Ductal carcinoma *in situ* (DCIS)**.

Internal mammary nodes Lymph nodes or glands sitting behind the breast-bone. Tissue fluid from the breast drains primarily to axillary lymph nodes but can also drain centrally to these nodes.

Invasive Spreading beyond usual boundaries. With breast cancer, this can refer to direct spread into surrounding tissues or more distant spread via lymphatic and/or blood vessels.

In-vitro fertilization (IVF) Production of an embryo—that is fertilization of an egg by sperm—taking place outside the body (i.e. in a test-tube).

Latissimus Dorsi (LD) reconstruction Breast reconstruction technique utilizing muscle, fat and skin from the back, often in conjunction with an implant for adequate bulk.

Lobular carcinoma *in situ* (LCIS) Abnormal but non-cancerous growth of cells lining the breast lobule (the milk-producing unit). Indicates a higher risk of future breast cancer.

Locally advanced breast cancer (LABC) Cancers which have any combination of the following: larger than 5cm, growing into skin, muscle or bone, causing other skin change such as **erythema** or **peau d'orange**.

Lumpectomy Surgical excision of a breast 'lump' or other lesion, which may be for diagnostic purposes or to alleviate symptoms. The breast is otherwise conserved. (Lumpectomy may be used in the context of breast-preserving cancer excision, although this should more properly be referred to as **wide local excision**.)

Lymph nodes/glands Glands within the lymphatic system which act as filtering or cleansing stations for **lymph** as it is ferried through the lymphatic vessels from the body's tissues back into the bloodstream.

Lymphoedema Chronic swelling of a body part due to inadequate removal of **lymph** by the lymphatic system. In breast cancer, lymphoedema most commonly affects the arm after surgery or radiotherapy to the axillary **lymph glands**.

Magnetic resonance imaging (MRI) Scan using a magnetic field rather than X-rays to produce internal pictures of the body. Increasingly used in screening for breast cancer in high-risk women as well as assessing more complicated breast cancers preoperatively.

Malignant Cancerous.

Mammogram Breast X-ray.

Margin The amount of normal tissue around a tumour in the surgical specimen.

Mastalgia Breast pain.

Mastectomy Surgical removal of all breast tissue on one side.

Medical oncologist Specialist who uses chemotherapy and other non-surgical therapies in the treatment on cancer.

Menarche The onset of menstruation—a female's first 'period'.

Menopause The cessation of menstrual periods—typically at around 50 years of age.

Metastasis/metastases Cancerous growths distant from the initial cancer.

Microarray technology A pathology technique which aims to make a 'fingerprint' of the molecular changes in a tissue.

Nausea Feeling of sickness with inclination to vomit.

Neo-adjuvant treatment Treatment such as chemotherapy, radiotherapy or hormonal therapy given prior to surgery in an attempt to make the latter more successful.

Neoplasm Abnormal growth of a tissue within the body. Can be **malignant** or **benign** (see above)

Nodal status Whether cancer has spread to nearby lymph nodes. In breast cancer, this usually refers to the status of the axillary nodes.

Oestrogen Hormone which promotes and maintains female characteristics.

Oestrogen receptor (ER) A molecule in the breast cancer cell that is 'switched on' by the attachment of oestrogen and may facilitate further growth/multiplication.

Oncologist Doctor specializing in cancer treatment.

Oophorectomy Surgical removal of the ovaries to reduce oestrogen levels by bringing forward menopause and/or to reduce the risk of ovarian cancer.

Open surgical biopsy Biopsy performed via a cut in the operating theatre. Surgical biopsy may be excisional (removing the entire lesion of interest) or incisional (removing a piece of a larger area of concern).

Osteoporosis A weakening of the bones that occurs with age and may be worsened by factors such as hormonal changes, lack of exercise and dietary imbalance.

Ovarian ablation Stopping of ovarian function either by removal at surgery or by radiotherapy. Irreversible.

Ovarian suppression Temporary cessation of ovarian function via administration of drugs such as the **gonadotrophin-releasing hormone (GnRH) analogues**.

Palliative care Treatment aimed at alleviating pain and other problems associated with an advanced and terminal disease state.

Palpable Detectable by touch.

PARP inhibitors An experimental therapy, which may be effective in treating BRCA and potentially other breast cancers. PARP means poly (ADP-ribose) polymerase and is involved in the repair of certain cells after damage.

Partial breast irradiation An experimental radiotherapy technique that aims to treat only the part of the breast affected by cancer.

Pathology The study of disease. Pathology can specifically refer to the type of disease within a given individual: 'Her pathology shows …'.

Peau d'orange French for 'the skin of an orange'. When the breast develops this swollen and discoloured appearance, it can be a sign of underlying cancer.

PET scans Full body scan looking for areas of high metabolism. Tumours are often revealed if they are metabolically very active.

Pre-invasive Cells which, whilst similar in appearance to invasive cancer cells, have not yet gained the ability to invade beyond their usual surrounds. See **Ductal carcinoma *in situ* (DCIS)** and *In situ*.

Progesterone Hormone which stimulates and regulates various female functions including menstruation and pregnancy.

Progesterone receptor (PgR) A molecule in the breast cancer cell that is 'switched on' by the attachment of progesterone and may facilitate further growth/multiplication.

Prognosis The likely outcome of a disease in an individual, based on outcomes of similar patients.

Prophylactic mastectomy Mastectomy performed when cancer is not present but to reduce the risk of it occurring by removing breast tissue pre-emptively.

Prosthesis Artificial body part such as an arm, leg or in the case of breast cancer, an artificial breast worn in the bra after mastectomy.

Radical or modified radical mastectomy Operations for breast cancer, involving removal of the breast as well as lymph glands from the axilla and in the 'radical' option, some chest muscles.

Radiotherapy Treatment of disease using radiation.

Recurrent cancer Relapse of cancer after a patient has been **disease-free** for a period.

Radiation oncologist Specialist who uses radiotherapy in the treatment on cancer.

Relapse See **Recurrent cancer**.

Remission Reduction in the severity of disease. Can be partial or complete and temporary or permanent.

Risk factor Something in a person's profile that increases his or her chances of developing a disease. In the context of breast cancer, risk factors include: a history in the family of breast cancer and a personal history of certain breast diseases.

Sentinel lymph node biopsy (SNB) Surgical biopsy of the first lymph gland/s the breast drains to in order to determine whether cancer has spread there, necessitating removal of further glands.

Seroma Collection of inflammatory fluid under the skin after surgery, which may require needle drainage intermittently.

Simple mastectomy Mastectomy without removal of any axillary lymph glands.

Skin-sparing or subcutaneous mastectomy Mastectomy with preservation of overlying skin +/– nipple and areola, for use in immediate **breast reconstruction**.

Staging Determination of the extent of cancer in the body.

Supraclavicular nodes Lymph glands in the area above the collarbone.

Survivorship The long-term issues for women following a diagnosis of cancer and the treatment for it.

Systemic treatment Treatments such as chemotherapy and hormonal therapy which are aimed at disease anywhere in the body, as opposed to surgery and radiotherapy which target specific areas where the disease load is greatest.

Tamoxifen Anti-oestrogen medication given daily, used in pre and postmenopausal women with hormone-sensitive breast cancers. It may also have a role in cancer prevention in some women.

Tissue expander Temporary expandable implant used in breast reconstruction surgery to gradually stretch up the tissues for the final implant, which is placed at a second operation.

Tissue flap Tissue taken from elsewhere in the body, for use in various functions at the disease site. See **Latissimus dorsi (LD) reconstruction** and **Transverse rectus abdominis muscle (TRAM) reconstruction**.

Tumour See **Neoplasm**.

Transverse rectus abdominis muscle (TRAM) reconstruction Breast reconstruction technique utilizing muscle, fat and skin from the abdomen.

Trastuzumab (Herceptin) see **Herceptin**.

Triple test Clinical (verbal and physical), radiological (mammogram, ultrasound, etc.) and histological (biopsy) assessment of concerning breast lesions, which is recommended to minimize the chance of missing cancer.

Ultrasound Method of radiologically assessing lesions within the body by the use of ultrasonic waves.

Wide local excision Surgical excision of a cancer as well as a margin of normal tissue around it. In breast cancer surgery, wide local excision is an alternative to mastectomy for smaller cancers.

Index